Pregnancy Nutrition

Good Health for You and Your Baby

70119102

Written for
The American Dietetic Association
by Elizabeth M. Ward, MS, RD

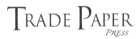

Trade Paper Press
An imprint of Turner Publishing Company
Nashville, Tennessee
www.turnerpublishing.com

Library of Congress Cataloging-in-Publication Data:

ISBN 0-471-34697-7

10 9 8 7 6

Pregnancy Nutrition

Good Health for You and Your Baby

Written for The American Dietetic Association by
Elizabeth M. Ward, MS, RD
Nutritionist, Harvard Vanguard
    Medical Associates
Boston, Massachusetts

The American Dietetic Association Reviewers:
Lorri Fishman, MS, RD
National Center for Nutrition
    and Dietetics

Maureen Murtaugh, PhD, RD
Rush Presbyterian St. Luke's
    Medical Center
Chicago, Illinois

Technical Editor:
Betsy Hornick, MS, RD
The American Dietetic Association
Chicago, Illinois

THE AMERICAN DIETETIC ASSOCIATION is the largest group of food and health professionals in the world. As the advocate of the profession, the ADA serves the public by promoting optimal nutrition, health, and well-being.

For expert answers to your nutrition questions, call the ADA/National Center for Nutrition and Dietetics Hot Line at (900) 225-5267. To listen to recorded messages or obtain a referral to a registered dietitian (RD) in your area, call (800) 366-1655. Visit the ADA's Website at www.eatright.org.

Contents

Introduction

YOU'RE PREGNANT! HOW WONDERFUL! As a mother-to-be, you've taken on your most important role ever. Expecting a child gives new meaning to eating a well-balanced diet, cutting out alcohol and smoking, and getting enough rest. In fact, your habits during pregnancy can influence your child for the rest of his life. Leading a healthy lifestyle is the best way to show your love for your growing baby.

The coming months will be filled with rapid growth—for both you and your baby—and changes that will bring excitement and joy, as well as fatigue, uncertainty, and apprehension. At times, you may feel as if you're riding a rollercoaster of emotions, happy one minute and down in the dumps the next. This is normal and quite common during pregnancy as you experience many physical and emotional changes and anticipate the life changes a new baby brings.

Pregnancy Nutrition was created to help make the eating right part of pregnancy easier. This essential guide is packed with practical advice. You'll learn what to eat for your growing baby and how to manage side effects of pregnancy. And you'll find answers to your many nutrition questions, presented in a simple, straightforward format.

While *Pregnancy Nutrition* helps you navigate healthy eating, it is not a substitute for the guidance of a qualified health care provider, such as a licensed physician, a certified nurse midwife, or perinatal nurse practitioner. Every pregnancy is unique, and pregnant women should visit their health care provider regularly, beginning early in pregnancy.

You've Just Found Out

Home pregnancy tests make finding out you're expecting quick, private, and convenient. Once you get a positive home pregnancy test reading, your doctor's office may ask you to have it confirmed by a more sophisticated blood test done through a laboratory or by another urine test in the doctor's office. Whatever the case, call your health care provider's office to schedule your first prenatal appointment after a positive home test.

Even with an appointment on the books, it can be weeks before you meet with your health care provider. What should you do in the meantime? Here are some suggestions to get you started on a healthy pregnancy.

➤ If you smoke, drink alcohol, or take any illicit drugs, stop now.
➤ Get plenty of rest.
➤ Exercise in moderation, not until exhaustion.
➤ If you're taking a multivitamin and mineral supplement that provides no more than 100 percent of the RDA for nutrients, it's fine to continue, but don't take any other supplement, such as extra vitamin C, or herbs. Your health care provider may prescribe a prenatal vitamin and mineral supplement before your first prenatal visit. If so, then stop taking the multivitamin.
➤ Eat a variety of foods and make sure that you are getting at least 400 micrograms of folic acid daily from fortified foods, vitamin supplements, or a combination of the two, in addition to the folate found naturally in certain foods. Folate is a B vitamin that can prevent neural tube defects, such as spina bifida, in your developing baby. Folic acid is the form of folate found in fortified foods and vitamin supplements. See page 17 for more on folate.
➤ Go easy on caffeine.
➤ Drink plenty of fluid, particularly water.

➤ Consult your doctor about any prescription or over-the-counter medications you are taking, or wish to take.

Test Your Pregnancy Nutrition Know-How

How much do you know about pregnancy nutrition? Find out with this simple quiz.

True or False?

1. You need to eat an extra 500 calories a day when pregnant.

2. It's not healthy to eat vegetarian during pregnancy.

3. Iron needs triple in pregnancy.

4. You should consume at least three servings of dairy foods daily when you're expecting, or the equivalent amount of calcium found in plant foods.

5. Most women should gain at least 25 pounds during pregnancy.

6. Pregnant women should stop exercising.

7. Snacking can lead to excessive weight gain in pregnancy.

8. Now that you're having a baby, you must give up your favorite high-fat fare.

9. Alcoholic beverages are not recommended in pregnancy.

10. A high-fiber diet is important during pregnancy.

Answers:

1. **False.** Pregnant women require 300 extra calories a day and nursing women need an extra 500 calories each day. You'll find more on calories and weight gain in Chapter 1 and nutrition tips while breast-feeding in Chapter 9.

2. **False.** With careful planning, a vegetarian eating style can be very healthy during pregnancy. If you're concerned, or if vegetarian eating is new to you, you'll want to consult a registered dietitian to ensure that you're meeting your nutrient needs. Read more about vegetarian eating during pregnancy in Chapter 8.

3. **False.** Your need for iron doubles during pregnancy. It can be difficult to get this much iron from food alone. That's why you should read more about iron in Chapter 3.

4. **True.** It's easy to meet your calcium requirements with at least three servings per day of dairy foods. Foods in the Milk, Cheese, and Yogurt Group supply an array of nutrients in addition to calcium. But calcium is also found in other foods, such as broccoli and calcium-fortified juices and cereals. Read more about calcium and its sources in Chapter 3, and serving guidelines for all five food groups in Chapter 5.

5. **True.** Most women should gain between 25 and 35 pounds, but each pregnancy and each woman is unique, so this recommendation is not set in stone. See Chapter 1 for more on healthy pregnancy weight gain.

6. **False.** While most women can continue with regular physical activity until close to delivery, some women must stop. See Chapter 6 to find out who cannot exercise when pregnant.

7. **False,** if you choose snacks wisely, **true,** if you don't. Snacking is a great way to get nutrients when it's done right. See Chapter 5 for snacking tips.

8. **False.** All foods can fit into a healthy diet, pregnant or not. Just don't overdo high-fat foods, such as chips and sweets. For more about fat, see Chapter 2.

9. **True.** Alcohol can have serious effects on a developing fetus. Read about alcohol and other fluids in Chapter 4.

10. **True.** Fiber helps prevent constipation, a common occurrence during pregnancy. Learn tips for managing constipation and other discomforts of pregnancy in Chapter 7.

Chapter One

Weight Gain
How Much is Enough?

LIKE MANY WOMEN, you've probably struggled with weight control, watching what you eat and working out regularly to stay fit. Along comes pregnancy, and the weight gain you took such pains to avoid before conceiving becomes paramount to your baby's health.

The health of your baby, and its weight at birth, are related to how much weight you gain during pregnancy. Your baby grows at a mind-boggling rate, 24 hours a day. Consider this: a growing fetus develops 100,000 brain cells a minute! And from about 26 weeks on, a fetus gains about an ounce of weight every day. That kind of growth takes a lot of energy. That's why pregnancy is no time to restrict calories.

Skimping on meals and snacks during pregnancy can pose serious risks for a growing baby. If you don't gain enough weight, you run the risk of having a low-birthweight baby, defined as 5 1/2 pounds or less. Low-birthweight babies have a greater chance of health problems and developmental difficulties.

Gaining too much weight as a mom-to-be has a downside, too. Babies born to moms who gain more than 35 pounds during pregnancy may face difficult delivery because they tend to be larger. Excessive weight gain also makes it harder for mom to lose pregnancy weight after giving birth.

Women pregnant with twins need to gain more weight. It makes sense that if you are having more than two babies, your weight gain goal would be even higher. Yet, little is known about how much weight gain is necessary when pregnant with three or more babies. That's why each woman should review her personal weight gain guidelines with her health care provider.

Weighing In on Pregnancy Gain

How much weight gain is enough for a healthy baby? That depends. The following are weight gain targets from the American College of Obstetricians and Gynecologists (ACOG). Keep in mind that these are only guidelines. Every pregnancy is unique, and so is every woman. For example, taller women, African American women, and teens may be advised to gain more. Ask your doctor what's right for you.

If you are...	Then gain...
Normal weight before conceiving	25 to 35 pounds
Overweight before conceiving	15 to 25 pounds
Underweight before conceiving	28 to 40 pounds
Carrying twins	35 to 45 pounds

Tracking Weight Gain

Your girth is expanding, and you're probably wondering where it's coming from. It may ease your mind to know what contributes to pregnancy weight gain.

	Approximate weight gain (lbs)
Baby	7 to 8
Placenta	1 to 2
Amniotic Fluid	2
Breasts	1
Uterus	2
Increase in blood volume	3
Body fat	5 or more
Increased muscle tissue and fluid	4 to 7
Total:	**At Least 25**

When can you expect weight gain to begin? Many women put on between 2 and 4 pounds in the first trimester, which lasts about 13 weeks. Some women may gain little or no weight in the first trimester because they aren't feeling well, while others gain more. Teens should aim for a 4 to 6 pound gain during the first three months of pregnancy.

Once the first trimester is over, weight gain should pick up, and become more steady. Aim for an average weight increase of 3/4 to 1 pound weekly from the second trimester on. Some months you may gain more, and some months less.

· ·

Is it OK...to give in to food cravings?

More than likely, yes. You will probably feel more hungry starting around your 13th week of pregnancy when estrogen, an appetite stimulant, begins rising in the bloodstream. It's generally OK to indulge your food cravings as long as they don't crowd out more nutritious foods or contribute to excessive weight gain.

· ·

Counting on Calories

Calories are the energy in food that your body harnesses to do its work. A full-term pregnancy requires about 80,000 calories. That may sound like a lot, but that number is deceiving. Consider that a full-term pregnancy is about 280 days (40 weeks). Spread out the total calories required for pregnancy and you need about 300 extra calories per day. Add this to an average energy requirement of 2,200 calories per day for women, and your calorie needs during pregnancy total about 2,500 a day. Of course, some women may need slightly more or less, depending on their age, activity level, and prepregnancy weight. For example, pregnant teens require more, as do very active women who may need as many as 2,900 calories daily.

Making Calories Count

Three hundred calories a day is not a lot to work with, so make them count. To get a variety of nutrients, choose foods from all five food groups, and make a variety of choices within each group. Here are some ways to "spend" about 300 calories:

➤ 2 cups (16 ounces) of 1% fat milk, and 2 ounces lean meat, poultry, or seafood

➤ 2 slices bread, 2 ounces tuna fish or turkey with 1 teaspoon reduced-fat mayonnaise

➤ 1 cup (8 ounces) of vanilla nonfat yogurt mixed with 1/2 cup fresh fruit and topped with 1 ounce crunchy cereal

Weight Gain

➤ 1 cup (8 ounces) skim or 1% low fat milk, and 1 slice whole wheat toast topped with 1 tablespoon peanut butter and 1 tablespoon raisins

Is it OK...to eat more frequently?

Yes, especially since many women find that small meals and snacks can help quell the nausea and fatigue experienced during pregnancy. As time goes on, smaller, more frequent meals may become a necessity as a growing baby crowds your stomach and intestines, making it hard to eat large meals. It doesn't matter whether you eat three meals, or divide your daily food intake into six or more mini-meals, as long as your servings from each food group total what you need for pregnancy. See Chapter 5 for more on food group servings.

Chapter Two

Fueling a Healthy Pregnancy

THE FUEL FOR a healthy pregnancy comes from carbohydrates, protein, and fat. Each of these nutrients provides calories and serves other important purposes. Eating a variety of foods makes it easy to meet your needs for carbohydrates, protein, and fat. No less vital to life—and a healthy baby—are vitamins, minerals, fiber, cholesterol, and water, which are not considered as "fuel" because they do not provide calories.

Carbohydrates

Most of your calories should come from carbohydrate-containing foods, such as bread, rice, pasta, fruits, and vegetables. Your body uses carbohydrates quickly and efficiently to meet energy demands. Fat is also used for energy but should not be your predominant calorie source.

If you don't consume enough calories to meet your energy needs, your body turns to protein for energy. Protein is an "expensive" source of energy because breaking down protein to meet energy needs diverts it from its many important functions. More about protein later.

To get enough carbohydrate in pregnancy, consume at least nine servings from the Bread, Cereal, Rice, and Pasta Group, at least three servings from the Fruit Group, and a minimum of three Vegetable Group selections. See Chapter 5 for more information on how to use Food Guide Pyramid guidelines during pregnancy.

Categorizing Carbohydrates

There are two carbohydrate categories, referred to as simple and complex. With the exception of fiber, all carbohydrates contain four calories per gram. Complex carbohydrates should dominate your diet as the primary energy source. Foods rich in complex carbohydrates are also packed with other nutrients. For example, a baked potato supplies ample amounts of B vitamins, vitamin C, potassium, and fiber, in addition to carbohydrate. And carbohydrate-packed, fortified breakfast cereals can be a source of many important nutrients, including iron and folate.

Table sugar is just one of several sugars referred to as simple carbohydrates. Table sugar (sucrose) is an added sugar in many different foods whereas the simple carbohydrates in fruit and fruit juices (fructose) and milk (lactose) are naturally occurring. While all provide the body with energy, the main differences between foods containing sucrose, fructose, and lactose are the accompanying nutrients.

Sugary, sweet foods, such as soda, candy, cookies, and cakes are tasty but typically serve up little in the way of nutrition. For example, sip 12 ounces of regular soda and you get nothing more than nearly 10 teaspoons of sugar and 150 calories. While 12 ounces of orange juice, as satisfyingly sweet, provides about the same calories as soda, it is also an excellent source of vitamin C and folate, both important vitamins during pregnancy. In addition, calcium-fortified orange juice can provide as much calcium as milk. So, should you trade in soda for juice when expecting? It's fine to drink juice, but be aware that drinking too much may cause excessive weight gain. Drink beverages such as water and milk to help meet most of your fluid needs. Read more about fluids in Chapter 4.

If you crave sweets, feast on fruit. Fruit is sweet and it has much to offer, including vitamins, minerals, and fiber—nutrients missing in cookies, cake, and candy. Other sweet treats, like frozen yogurt, ice cream, and pudding, provide protein, vitamins, and minerals, making them wise choices, too.

Fiber: A Complex Issue

Fiber is a component of plant foods. Like other complex carbohydrates, fiber keeps good company. It's found in foods typically packed with vitamins and minerals, including grains, vegetables, and fruits. But it's also different from its carbohydrate counterparts in that your body cannot digest it. That's why fiber contributes no calories.

One of fiber's benefits during pregnancy is that it can help alleviate constipation and hemorrhoids that expectant women often experience. Fiber softens and adds bulk to stools, stimulating your intestines to pass them faster and with greater ease. When you strain to move your bowels, hemorrhoids can develop. That's why avoiding constipation is key to warding off hemorrhoids.

Fiber and fluid are essential partners. Fiber absorbs many times its weight in fluid, so sipping at least eight glasses of non-caffeinated fluid daily, including water, milk, and juice, enhances fiber's beneficial effects. Regular physical activity also helps relieve constipation because it increases blood flow to the intestine, helping to keep digestion running smoothly.

Focus on Fiber

Pregnant or not, you need 20 to 35 grams of fiber every day. Fiber is supplied by whole grain foods, fruits, vegetables, legumes, nuts, and seeds. Making these foods regular choices helps to meet your fiber needs. Here's how to get your fill of fiber.

Food	Fiber (grams)
Breads, Grains, Pasta	
Pumpernickel bread, 1 slice	3
Whole wheat bread, 1 slice	2
Brown rice, cooked, 1/2 cup	2
Spaghetti, cooked, 1/2 cup	1
Cereals	
100% bran, 1/3 cup	8
Bran flakes, 3/4 cup	5
Raisin bran, 3/4 cup	5
Oatmeal, cooked, 3/4 cup	3
Fruit	
Pear, with skin, 1 medium	4
Figs, dried, 2	4
Strawberries, 1 cup	4

Food	Fiber (grams)
Apple, with skin, 1 medium	3
Orange, 1 medium	3
Banana, 1 medium	2
Vegetables	
Potato, baked, with skin, 1 medium	4
Sweet potato, baked with skin, 1 medium	4
Brussel sprouts, 1/2 cup, cooked	3
Broccoli, 1/2 cup, cooked	2
Peas, 1/2 cup, cooked	2
Carrots, raw, 1 medium	2
Tomato, raw, 1 medium	2
Legumes, cooked	
Garbanzo beans, 1/2 cup	6
Kidney beans, 1/2 cup	3
Lentils, 1/2 cup	4
Baked beans, 1/2 cup	3
Nuts and seeds	
Peanuts, dry roasted, 1/4 cup	3
Sunflower seeds, 1/4 cup	3
Walnuts, 1/4 cup	1

Is it OK...to eat foods with artificial sweeteners when expecting?

Yes, in moderation. All of the intense (artificial) sweeteners approved by the Food and Drug Administration (FDA)—aspartame, saccharin, and acesulfame-K—are considered safe during pregnancy. But pregnancy is no time to cut calories, so the best approach is to meet your serving goals from the Food Guide Pyramid first and then include foods with non-nutritive sweeteners if you still feel hungry. Also keep in mind that foods made with artificial sweeteners, such as diet soda, are often lacking in essential nutrients needed for pregnancy. Pregnant women with the rare genetic disorder phenylketonuria (PKU) should not eat foods made with aspartame, because they cannot break down phenylalanine, one of aspartame's components.

Protein

Moms-to-be need protein to make new cells, manufacture enzymes and hormones that regulate life, and control fluid balance. In a pinch, protein can also be used as a source of energy, since it provides four calories per gram. With its important responsibilities, it's clear why protein is paramount during pregnancy.

Most Americans eat more than enough protein, which is found in both animal and plant foods. But some women skimp on protein, especially if watching calories. Why? Many protein-packed foods, such as meat, poultry, eggs, and full-fat dairy products, also contain fat. Weight-conscious women may cut back on these foods to limit fat and calories.

If that sounds familiar, check the following chart, Protein Power, to tally your daily protein grams and to look for protein-packed foods you can include in your pregnancy diet. Or you could simply eat at least 6 ounces of meat, poultry, or seafood (or their equivalents) daily and consume at least three dairy product servings daily to meet your protein needs. See Chapter 5 for food group serving information.

Pregnant women need 60 grams of protein every day. That's about 10 extra grams of protein each day. It's particularly important to get adequate protein from food, because protein is not provided in prenatal supplements and because high protein foods have so much to offer in the way of nutrients. For example, milk supplies not only protein but vitamin D, calcium, and phosphorus—all necessary for building strong bones in baby and mother. Likewise, meat, poultry, and seafood contain iron, necessary to transport oxygen to a growing baby.

Protein Power

Getting enough protein? Check your eating pattern against the chart.

Food	Calories	Protein (grams)
Beef, extra lean, roasted, 3 ounces	150	25
Bread, whole wheat, 1 slice	70	3
Bulgur, cooked, 1 cup	150	6
Cereal, ready-to-eat, bran flakes, 3/4 cup	95	3
Cereal, cream of wheat, 3/4 cup cooked	100	3

Food	Calories	Protein (grams)
Cheese, 1 ounce		
Cheddar	115	7
Part-skim mozzarella	70	7
Chicken, roasted, 3 ounces		
White meat, no skin	150	27
Dark meat, no skin	175	23
Cottage cheese, 1 cup, 1% low fat	165	28
Egg, 1 large, whole	75	6
Egg white, 1 large	15	3
Garbanzo beans, cooked, 1 cup	285	12
Lentils, boiled, 1 cup	230	18
Lobster, cooked, 3 ounces	85	17
Milk, 8 ounces		
Whole	150	8
Skim	85	8
Pasta, enriched, cooked, 1 cup	190	6
Peanut butter, 2 tablespoons	190	9
Pizza, cheese, 4 ounce slice	280	15
Pork, top loin, broiled, 3 ounces	175	26
Salmon, Atlantic, cooked, 3 ounces	155	22
Tofu, raw, 1/2 cup	95	10
Tuna, white, drained, 3 ounces	115	23
Wheat germ, 1/4 cup	105	7
Yogurt, low fat, fruited, 8 ounces	225	9

· ·

Is it OK...to avoid eating meat while pregnant?

Meat, including beef, pork, poultry, and lamb, is rich in protein, vitamins, and minerals, including iron and zinc. If you suddenly develop an aversion to meat, or if you never had a taste for it, don't worry. Make sure you get adequate protein from other sources, such as dairy products, legumes, nuts, and grain foods, and eat a wide array of nutritious foods from all the food groups to obtain other nutrients like iron that you're missing by excluding meat. Read more about vegetarian eating in Chapter 8.

· ·

Fat

Have you ever counted fat grams? Chances are you have at one time. At 9 calories per gram, many women take pains to limit fat intake when striving for weight control.

Fat is an essential nutrient, whether pregnant or not. But fat is particularly important when you're expecting. As the sole provider of essential fatty acids, dietary fat is pivotal in the proper development of baby's brain and central nervous system. Equally important to pregnancy is fat's role in transporting the vitamins A, D, E, and K—all necessary for healthy babies. Last but not least, fat is a concentrated energy source, helping provide the calories you need to foster baby's growth.

How much fat is enough? Health professionals recommend limiting fat calories to 30 percent or less of you total intake. Since your primary goals during pregnancy are to meet your calorie and protein needs, fat restriction should not be a major concern. But don't go overboard on fat either. Balance high-fat favorites with low-fat fare to increase eating satisfaction, eliminate feelings of deprivation, and provide the nutrients you need to nurture baby.

What's the best fat? All types of fats contain more than twice the calories of carbohydrate or protein. Most fats, such as olive oil, vegetable oil, margarine, and butter, contain about 120 calories and 13 grams of fat per tablespoon. Since they all contain about the same number of calories, which type of fat should you eat?

Polyunsaturated and monounsaturated fats are considered the healthiest because of their effect on blood cholesterol level. Even though blood cholesterol concentrations rise as a result of pregnancy, the bulk of your fat intake should come from these two heart-healthy types, when you're expecting and afterward.

Monounsaturated fat is the predominant fat in foods such as olive oil, avocado, peanuts, peanut butter, and other nuts. Cooking oils, such as safflower, sunflower, and corn, and tub margarines are rich in polyunsaturated fat, and contain smaller amounts of monounsaturated and saturated fat, too.

Seafood supplies a type of polyunsaturated fat known as omega-3. Omega-3 fatty acids help build your baby's brain and eye tissue. To get more omega-3 fat, include fish in your diet regularly, especially the fattier varieties, such as salmon and bluefish.

Too much saturated fat may increase blood cholesterol levels. Animal foods, including full-fat dairy products, fatty meat, poultry skin, chocolate, and butter, are sources of saturated fat. Hydrogenated fat, used in food processing, is another form of saturated fat that you may see on food ingredient labels. When cooking oils are hydrogenated for storage or cooking purposes, their polyunsaturated and monounsaturated fatty acids are converted into more saturated forms. Hydrogenated fat is found in processed foods including margarine, commercially baked goods, fried foods, and snack foods.

Lower-Fat Eating Tips

Even though pregnancy is no time to drastically restrict fat intake, choosing more fresh and lightly processed foods helps keep fat intake in control without compromising taste and nutrition. Here are some tips.

➤ Eat lean meat, skinless poultry, and seafood more often. Trim the fat from meat and the skin from poultry before cooking.

➤ Opt for reduced-fat and fat-free dairy products. You'll skimp on fat, not nutrition.

➤ Offset high-fat food choices with low-fat fare. If you crave ice cream, go ahead and indulge. Just balance this with lower-fat food choices.

➤ Trade in traditional toppings. For example, replace cream cheese on your bagel with 1/4 cup of nutrient-packed low-fat cottage cheese, and replace butter or sour cream on your baked potato with an herb-flavored yogurt.

➤ If you snack regularly on cookies or chips, try alternating this with fresh fruits and vegetables to help satisfy your need for sweet or crunchy foods.

➤ Go for the least-processed foods possible. For example, French fries contain about 30 times the fat of baked potatoes.

Is it OK...to have fat substitutes when expecting?

Yes, but remember that fat is vital to proper growth and development of your growing baby. It's true that fat-modified foods, such as reduced-fat chips and frozen desserts, can help keep fat in control, but many fat-reduced foods contain as many, if not more, calories because sugar is often added to make up for the flavor lost with the fat. Food manufacturers use a variety of methods to cut fat without compromising taste and satisfaction. Some fat replacers are derived from carbohydrates, some are protein-based, while others are made from fats.

Chapter Three

Vitamins
and Minerals
The Supporting Cast

Vital Vitamins

Carbohydrate, protein, and fat may be the fuel for pregnancy, but they wouldn't amount to anything without the spark supplied by vitamins. Vitamins regulate the metabolism, digestion, and absorption of the three calorie-containing nutrients and oversee many other bodily functions that keep you healthy and your baby's growth on track.

Vitamins are divided into two classes: fat-soluble and water-soluble. Vitamins A, D, E, and K travel and dissolve in fat. Fat-soluble vitamins from food are stored in your liver and fat tissue and are used as needed. The B vitamins and vitamin C dissolve in water. Because your body cannot store water-soluble vitamins, it's important that when pregnant you get enough B vitamins and vitamin C on most days.

The most notable vitamins needed during pregnancy are highlighted here.

Vitamin A

If you see vitamin A as necessary for good eyesight, your "vision" is 20–20. But vitamin A is also an all-around nutrient that makes possible the growth and health of cells and tissues throughout the body.

The daily requirement for adult women is 5,000 International Units (I.U.), whether pregnant or not. You should make sure you get enough, but not too much. While vitamin A is essential, more than the RDA may be harmful. Large doses of vitamin A obtained from supplements (10,000 I.U. and higher) can cause birth defects.

Vitamin A is found in both animal and plant foods. Animal products contain the pre-formed form of vitamin A called retinol. Fruits and vegetables contain carotenoids, substances the body converts into vitamin A. Excellent sources of vitamin A include:

➤ Sweet potato
➤ Carrots
➤ Spinach
➤ Milk (most of which is vitamin A fortified)
➤ Liver

Vitamin D

Vitamin D fosters calcium absorption from food and helps deposit calcium into bones, making them dense and strong. Pregnancy does not increase your vitamin D requirement, which remains at 200 International Units (I.U.) per day for women under age 50.

Vitamin D is one of the few vitamins your body can make. Sunlight sparks the process in your skin, which is finished off in your liver and kidneys. Your body can use vitamin D right away or store it for later. Healthy people who get regular sun exposure can make enough vitamin D to last the whole year. The problem is, many women don't get adequate exposure to the strong ultraviolet rays needed to make vitamin D because they live in northern climates where the sun is strong enough for only about half the year. And wearing sunscreens with a sun protection factor (SPF) of 8 or higher blocks most of the rays that initiate vitamin D production. That's why it's important to rely on food for vitamin D. With the exception of foods such as eggs and salmon with bones, few foods naturally contain vitamin D. Fortunately, some frequently consumed foods are fortified with vitamin D, including:

➤ Milk
➤ Margarine
➤ Breakfast cereals (check the Nutrition Facts panel)

B Vitamins

The B vitamins are a complex of vitamins with closely-related functions. You need more B vitamins when pregnant because these important vitamins are involved in releasing and using the energy in food. B vitamins are easy to find in most of the food groups. The only food groups not particularly rich in B vitamins are the Fruit and the Vegetable Groups.

B vitamin	Function	Pregnancy requirement	Food sources
Thiamin (B_1)	Releases energy from carbohydrate	1.4 milligrams	Pork, whole grain and enriched grain products, lentils
Riboflavin (B_2)	Helps produce energy; helps in protein use	1.4 milligrams	Dairy products, organ meats, enriched grains
Niacin (B_3)	General metabolism, particularly use of carbohydrate and fat	18 milligrams	Meat, poultry, seafood, nuts, fortified grains
Pyridoxine (B_6)	Helps body in making proteins used to make cells	1.9 milligrams	Poultry, fish, pork, bananas
Vitamin B_{12}	Helps make red blood cells along with folate; helps in using fat and carbohydrates	2.6 micrograms	Found mostly in animal foods, with the exception of some nutritional yeast products and fortified soy milk and cereal

Folate

Folate is vital for producing new and healthy red blood cells. Over time, too little folate leads to a blood disorder called megaloblastic anemia where underdeveloped blood cells are unable to carry adequate oxygen. What's worse is that folate deficiency may cause neural tube defects (NTDs), a serious birth defect that occurs early in pregnancy—often before a woman suspects she's pregnant. Recently released recommendations for folate advise that any woman capable of becoming pregnant (14–50 years) should get 400 micrograms of folic acid daily from foods fortified with folic acid, from vitamin supplements, or a combination of the two. This is in addition to the folate found naturally in certain foods. Folic acid is the form of folate found in fortified foods and dietary supplements.

Beginning in January 1998, enriched grain products, including most breads, flour, pastas, rice, and cereals, are required by law to be fortified with folic acid. On the labels of these fortified products, you'll see folate (or folic acid) listed on the Nutrition Facts panel along with its % Daily Value (% DV). The % DV tells you how a serving of the food contributes to your daily needs. To meet your daily requirement of 400 micrograms, the % DV for folate (or folic acid) from your food choices and vitamin supplements over the course of a day should add up to at least 100%. Keep in mind that the only foods that contain folate in the form of folic acid are fortified grain products.

Since it is so important to get enough folate even before you know you're pregnant, it may pay to take a multivitamin and mineral supplement—especially if you suspect that you're not getting enough from foods fortified with folic acid. Once you know you're pregnant, the folate requirement for pregnancy increases to 600 micrograms per day. It's important that at least 400 micrograms come from fortified foods or supplements, and the remaining 200 micrograms can come from foods with naturally occurring folate. Most prenatal vitamins meet the requirements for folic acid, but you'll also need to include more folate from your food choices.

Food	Approx. Folate (micrograms)
Lentils, cooked, 1 cup	358
Spinach, cooked, 1 cup	263
Chickpeas, cooked, 1 cup	160
Orange juice, made from frozen concentrate, 1 cup	109
Peas, cooked, 1 cup	101
Ready-to-eat cereal, 1 ounce	100–400*
Pasta, 1/2 cup	100–120*
Oatmeal, instant, 1/2 cup	80*
Rice, 1/2 cup	60*
Spinach, raw, 1 cup	58
Bread, 1 slice	40*
Broccoli, cooked, 1/2 cup	39
Strawberries, raw, sliced, 1 cup	26
Orange, 1, medium	24

*These fortified foods contain folic acid.

Vitamin C

Most people associate vitamin C with fighting off colds and flu. While vitamin C is necessary for a healthy immune system, when it comes to building a healthy baby, vitamin C has many more important functions. Among its talents: vitamin C aids in the production of collagen, a cement-like substance that provides structure to the body by holding together bones and tissues; it helps keep blood vessels strong; and it promotes the formation and repair of red blood cells and healthy gums. On top of that, vitamin C helps you absorb more iron found in some plant foods, such as grains and vegetables, so try to include at least one vitamin C source at most meals.

You need 70 milligrams of vitamin C a day during pregnancy, which is 10 milligrams more per day than for nonpregnant women. Foods rich in vitamin C include:

➤ Orange juice
➤ Red bell pepper
➤ Orange
➤ Kiwi
➤ Tomato
➤ Strawberries
➤ Grapefruit

Making the Most of Vitamins

Buy the freshest foods possible, and treat them with care. For the most nutrition, purchase robust-looking fruits and vegetables or their high-quality frozen counterparts.

Choose milk in opaque containers and refrigerate it immediately after using to better preserve nutrients like riboflavin and vitamin A, which are lessened by light.

Eat raw fruits and vegetables more often. Even proper cooking will destroy some vitamins, especially heat-sensitive ones like vitamin C and folate.

If you cook fruits and vegetables, preserve their nutrients by steaming quickly in a covered pot or by microwaving. Cook produce only until crisp, not mushy.

Eat the skin of fruits and vegetables when possible. Peel away edible skins and you toss nutrients. Wash produce thoroughly and enjoy.

There's no need to rinse most grains, such as rice and pasta, before or after cooking. You're just washing away nutrition.

●●●

Must-Have Minerals

Like vitamins, minerals help orchestrate many processes in your body. As a group, the mighty minerals are versatile: they ferry oxygen, normalize heartbeat, and make for strong bones and teeth, among many other functions.

Calcium

Calcium is the body's most abundant mineral. A mom-to-be needs enough calcium during pregnancy to meet her own needs as well as what baby needs to construct his healthy bones and teeth. A small but critical fraction of total body calcium circulates in the bloodstream to aid cell function and nerve transmission, and to maintain a normal heartbeat.

Nearly all calcium is stored in bones, making them your calcium "bank account." Your baby gets the calcium he needs from your bones, and vitamin D helps facilitate the transfer. To make up for baby's calcium "withdrawal," hormones help you absorb more calcium from food, and deposit it in your bones. In fact, pregnant women may absorb nearly twice the calcium of their nonpregnant counterparts.

Even with the boost in absorption, you need a steady supply of dietary calcium to satisfy the demands pregnancy puts on your calcium stores. If you don't get enough calcium with each pregnancy, and between, you could be at risk for osteoporosis, a crippling bone disease that causes bones to become brittle and increases your risk of bone fractures later in life.

Pregnant women require 1,000 milligrams (mg) of calcium each day. To get that much, health professionals recommend consuming at least three to four servings a day from the Milk, Yogurt, and Cheese Group, or by consuming the equivalent amount from plant foods. Dairy products are excellent calcium sources. Milk, regardless of fat or lactose content, is particularly beneficial for pregnant women because it contains calcium and vitamin D, as well as other minerals needed for good health.

Plant foods may contain substances that reduce calcium absorption, as in the case of spinach, Swiss chard, and wheat bran. Still, calcium-fortified plant-based foods, such as some juices, soy milk, and bread products, can provide substantial calcium. Just read the labels carefully to find products that are calcium-fortified.

Calcium Countdown
Calcium is found in many foods, but dairy foods dominate. Add up your daily calcium intake with this chart.

Food	Portion size	Approximate Calcium (mg)
Caffe latte	12 ounces	410
Yogurt, fruit	8 ounces	315
Milk, all types	8 ounces	300

Food	Portion size	Approximate Calcium (mg)
Chocolate milk, 2% fat	8 ounces	285
Calcium-fortified soy milk	8 ounces	250–300
Cappuccino	12 ounces	260
Swiss cheese	1 ounce	270
Tofu (processed with calcium sulfate)	1/2 cup	260
Orange juice, calcium-fortified	3/4 cup	225
Cheese pizza	1/8 of a 15-inch pizza	220
Cheddar cheese	1 ounce	205
Salmon, canned with edible bones	3 ounces	205
Molasses, blackstrap	1 tablespoon	170
Mozzarella cheese, part-skim	1 ounce	185
Frozen yogurt	1/2 cup	105
Turnip greens, cooked	1/2 cup	100
Dry milk powder	1 tablespoon	95
Ice cream	1/2 cup	85
Cottage cheese	1/2 cup	75
Parmesan cheese	1 tablespoon	70
Okra	1/2 cup	50
Orange	1	50
Broccoli, cooked	1/2 cup	45

Is it OK...to take calcium supplements?

If you can't get enough calcium from your food choices, a supplement may be a good idea. But first seek the advice of your health care provider or a registered dietitian (R.D.). A dietitian can assess your overall diet and calcium intake, and determine the type and amount of calcium supplements you should take, if any. If prescribed a calcium supplement, here's what to keep in mind. It's best to take calcium supplements with meals and to avoid any with added vitamin D, since too much vitamin D can harm a developing baby. Split up your calcium dose, too, taking no more than 500 milligrams at a time to improve absorption and reduce the risk of constipation. If you take both calcium and iron supplements, take them at different times of the day; they'll each be better absorbed. And never take calcium supplements made from bone meal, oyster shell, or dolomite, since they may contain contaminants like lead.

Do you ditch dairy? If you have bloating, gas, and diarrhea after devouring dairy foods, you may be lactose intolerant. This means you cannot break down lactose, the carbohydrate found in milk, because you lack adequate lactase. Lactase is the intestinal enzyme responsible for lactose digestion.

Chances are you can tolerate lactose-reduced foods, such as Lactaid brand milk. Over-the-counter drops of the enzyme lactase can be added to foods like milk, yogurt, or pudding to lower lactose levels. Tablets containing lactase can be consumed along with other lactose-containing foods, such as pizza, lasagna, and milk-based soups.

Luckily, lactose intolerance is not an all-or-nothing affair. You may be able to tolerate more lactose than you think. It's a matter of experimenting to find out how much lactose bothers you. Try these tricks to help improve your tolerance of lactose-containing foods:

➤ Drink milk with food. For example, cereal with milk or milk and a sandwich.

➤ Opt for lower-lactose foods. Try American, cheddar, Swiss, and Parmesan cheeses, yogurt, and buttermilk.

➤ Eat small portions of high-lactose foods in a sitting, such as 4 ounces of milk instead of 8 or 12.

➤ Choose higher-fat dairy foods, such as 2% reduced-fat or whole milk, and most regular cheeses. Fat can improve tolerance to lactose.

Allergic to milk? If your doctor has diagnosed a milk allergy, then by all means avoid dairy products. If you only suspect you're allergic to milk, you may be surprised to find out how rare milk allergies are in adults. Surveys suggest that approximately a third of adults think they are allergic to food, but true food allergy affects less than 2 percent of the adult population.

A food allergy involves the body's immune system, which is the main difference between food allergy and intolerance. If you are allergic to food, your body regards certain food components as invaders and tries to defend itself by releasing histamine and other chemicals. Symptoms of food allergy include hives, breathing problems, vomiting, and diarrhea. In some cases, food allergies can lead to death. Peanuts, milk, eggs, wheat, soy, tree nuts (almonds, walnuts, pecans), fish, and shellfish are the foods most likely to cause food allergy distress. If you suspect food allergy, consult an allergist.

Disguising Dairy

Don't like dairy foods "straight up"? Here are some hints for hiding them:

Prepare canned soups, such as tomato, with milk instead of water.

Whip up a fruit smoothie in your blender with milk or yogurt, calcium-fortified orange juice, fruit, and ice (see page 76).

Mash potatoes with evaporated milk, which contains twice the calcium of regular milk.

Enjoy dairy-based treats, such as pudding and frozen yogurt, for snacks.

Cook with dairy products.

Skip the sour cream, and make dips with plain yogurt instead.

Add dry milk powder to hot chocolate mix, instant hot cereal, or milk-based soups, such as tomato. Each tablespoon adds 95 milligrams of calcium, the equivalent of 1/3 glass fluid milk.

••

Iron

A developing baby requires lots of oxygen. What does that have to do with iron? Iron is involved in hemoglobin production. Hemoglobin is the portion of baby's and mom's red blood cells that carries oxygen and makes it available to cells. Iron also promotes a healthy immune system and plays a role in energy production.

Your iron needs double in pregnancy to 30 milligrams (mg) a day, an amount that can be tough to meet through food. In addition, some women begin pregnancy with poor iron stores due to monthly blood loss coupled with low-iron diets. So when baby's iron demands increase, beginning in the second trimester, many expectant women experience iron-deficiency anemia. That's when your health care provider may prescribe additional iron in the form of a supplement. Many prenatal supplements also contain adequate iron. Be aware, though, that iron supplements can cause an unpleasant side effect of constipation, especially if your fiber intake is low. Read about how to boost your fiber intake on page 7. Nausea can also be a side effect of iron supplements.

Even if you take an iron supplement, make an effort to include food sources of iron to ensure your body is absorbing enough. Food iron comes in two forms: heme, found mostly in animal foods, and non-heme, present primarily in plant foods but found in animal foods, too. Heme iron is better absorbed by the body than nonheme iron, even though foods with nonheme iron may actually contain more iron. Consuming vitamin C-rich foods with meals helps to boost nonheme iron absorption, as does eating animal sources of iron, such as beef, and iron-containing plant foods, such as a baked potato, at the same meal. Because substances called polyphenols in coffee or tea decrease nonheme iron uptake by the body, it's best to drink coffee or tea between meals.

Here are some ideas for boosting your iron intake and enhancing its absorption:

➤ Eat a vitamin-C rich food, such as orange juice, tomatoes, strawberries, and grapefruit, with iron-rich plant foods, such as whole grains, legumes, and fortified breakfast cereals, at the same meal or snack.

➤ Combine foods with heme and nonheme iron. For example, pair up hamburger (primarily heme iron) with an iron-enriched bun (nonheme iron).

➤ Avoid coffee and tea with meals. Wait two hours after your meal to enjoy coffee and tea, including decaffeinated versions.

Iron-Clad Foods

Food	Portion	Approximate Iron (mg)
Mostly Heme Iron		
Beef, tenderloin, broiled	3 ounces	3.1
Beef, sirloin, lean, broiled	3 ounces	2.9
Shrimp, cooked	3 ounces	2.6
Tuna, light meat, canned	3 ounces	1.3
Chicken, breast, roasted, white meat, skinless	3 ounces	1.0
Pork, lean, roasted	3 ounces	1.0
Non-Heme Iron		
Fortified breakfast cereal	1/2 cup	about 2–9*
Molasses, blackstrap	1 tablespoon	3.5
Spinach, boiled	1/2 cup	3.2
Potato, baked, with skin	1 medium	2.8
Red kidney beans, cooked	1/2 cup	2.6
Enriched rice, cooked	1/2 cup	1.2
Raisins, seedless	1/3 cup	1.1
Whole wheat bread	1 slice	0.9

*Products vary. Check Nutrition Facts label.

Sodium

When you think sodium, you may think swell, as in "swell up." True, sodium helps your body hold on to water, but that's critical for maintaining normal blood pressure, especially during pregnancy. This much-maligned mineral is also needed for normal muscle contraction and nerve conduction.

The minimum pregnancy sodium requirement is about 570 milligrams (mg) of sodium daily; during breastfeeding it's 635. Don't worry about getting these minimal amounts. Most women easily consume far more.

Sodium is a component of most foods, whether it occurs naturally or is added. Most of the sodium we consume comes from processed and prepared foods, such as fast food, canned products, and snacks, including chips. Sodium is a component of salt, but it is also found in food additives, including monosodium glutamate (MSG), sodium citrate, and disodium phosphate, used in many processed and prepared products.

You shouldn't forego sodium when you're pregnant. But neither should you go overboard. Aim for about 3,000 milligrams of sodium a day, but know that more on some days is acceptable. Over time, a consistently high sodium intake can interfere with calcium absorption. Read the Nutrition Facts panel to help monitor how much sodium you're getting from packaged foods. A healthy pregnancy diet is naturally low in sodium because it is based on fresh and lightly-processed foods, including fresh fruits and vegetables and whole grain products.

Seeking Sodium Sources
Sodium lurks in many foods. Do you know how much you're getting?

Food	Approximate sodium (mg)
Salt, 1 teaspoon	2,300
Fast food grilled chicken caesar salad	1,170
Soy sauce, 1 tablespoon	1,030
Tomato juice, 1 cup	875
Chicken noodle soup, chunky, ready-to-serve, 1 cup	850
Ham, deli style, 2 ounces	745
Peas, canned, 1/2 cup	215

About Vitamin and Mineral Supplements
Without question, good nutrition is based on a well-balanced diet, not dietary supplements. Food and its nutrients have much to offer a developing baby. If you eat a variety of foods and take time to plan your food choices, it is possible to fulfill most of your pregnancy vitamin and mineral needs with food. There is

no need to worry if you don't eat the perfect pregnancy diet every day, as long as your nutrient needs are met over the course of a few days. But when women regularly avoid certain foods and food groups, nutrient deficiencies that affect baby's development can result. That's why your health care provider may prescribe a prenatal multivitamin and mineral supplement.

However, not all health professionals agree that pregnant women need a multivitamin and mineral supplement for a healthy baby, although a daily iron supplement is usually prescribed for pregnant women beginning in the second trimester to meet increased iron needs that can be difficult to meet by food alone. A supplement containing at least 400 micrograms of folic acid, a form of the B vitamin folate, may also be warranted. While you should strive to get most of your nutrients from food first, prescribed prenatal pills pose little if any risk to mother or baby, and offer an inexpensive "security blanket" with benefits that may be great. Just remember, supplements can't make up for unhealthy lifestyle choices or for overall poor food choices.

A word of warning: Just because a little is good, more is not better when it comes to vitamins and minerals in pregnancy. That's why you should take only what your health care provider recommends.

Some women find swallowing big pills problematic, and others experience nausea after taking a prenatal supplement. If these are problems for you, try these tips:

➤ Ask your health care provider or pharmacist if it is OK to cut the supplement in half. Then take half in the morning and the other half at night.

➤ Take your supplement with food.

➤ Take your supplement before you go to bed with a small snack.

➤ Keep in mind that iron is absorbed best on an empty stomach. So if you're able, take the entire pill at night on an empty stomach.

Is it OK...to take herbal supplements when pregnant?

To play it safe, no. Echinacea to fight colds, feverfew to ward off migraines, and St. John's wort to thwart depression are attractive alternatives when most traditional medications are off-limits in pregnancy. But herbal remedies should be regarded as drugs, even though they are regulated as dietary supplements in the United States. In addition, simply being plant-based does not make a remedy safe, during pregnancy or not. For example, herbal teas and supplements made from comfrey can be toxic to the liver. Pennyroyal stimulates uterine contractions and should never be consumed by a pregnant woman.

Chapter Four

What's to Drink?

WATER IS THE forgotten nutrient, yet it's the most indispensable of all. Without water, you'd survive just a few days, and your pregnancy would be in peril. Water helps your body cool off; transports nutrients and waste products; moistens the digestive tract and tissues; and cushions and protects your developing baby.

Fluids for Two

Fluid needs increase when pregnant, in part to keep up with an expanding blood supply, the bulk of which is water. Pregnancy requires at least 64 ounces (eight 8-ounce cups) of fluid each day. Water is the most obvious fluid source, and often the most desirable, because it is rapidly absorbed by the body. Milk, juice, and noncaffeinated soft drinks also count toward satisfying fluid needs because they contain water. So do certain solid foods, such as fruits and vegetables.

Caffeinated beverages, including coffee, tea, and soft drinks, cause your body to lose water and should not be counted toward fluid intake. Regular soft drinks are high in sugar and devoid of nutrients, and many also contain caffeine, so use them sparingly. Take it easy on juice, too. Juice is healthy, but it has almost as many calories as regular soft drinks.

Fluid Foods

As you may have guessed, fruits and vegetables contain the most water; fatty foods have the least.

Food	Percent Water by Weight
Lettuce	95
Tomato	94
Broccoli, cooked	91
Orange	86
Apricot	86
Apple	85
Banana	76
Bread, white	36
Cookie	5
Vegetable oil	0

Water With a Twist

Sip on these variations of a glass of water:

Add lemon, lime, or orange slices to a pitcher of water, and keep in refrigerator.

Mix 6 ounces club soda or seltzer with a splash of orange juice or lemonade.

Make iced tea with your favorite herbal tea bags.

Lowdown on Caffeine

Should pregnant women consume caffeine? There's little reliable scientific evidence linking caffeine to miscarriage or birth defects, yet caffeine remains a source of debate among health professionals.

Whatever caffeine's effects, one thing's for sure: caffeine causes your body to lose water and can lead to dehydration. Going easy on regular coffee, tea, and caffeine-containing soda (read the ingredient label since non-cola soft drinks may contain caffeine) will help ensure that your body is able to absorb enough fluids. Caffeine pops up in other less "obvious" foods, too. One cup of some coffee-flavored frozen desserts and yogurt contain more caffeine than 12 ounces of cola.

A reasonable caffeine limit for pregnant and breast-feeding

women appears to be 300 milligrams (mg) or less daily. The Nutrition Facts label does not state caffeine content, but this chart can help you count caffeine:

Food or Beverage	Caffeine (mg)	
	Typical Amount	Range
Coffee, 8 ounces		
Brewed, drip method	100	60–180
Instant	65	30–120
Decaffeinated	3	1–5
Espresso coffee (single, 2-ounce serving)	100	40–170
Tea, 8 ounces		
Brewed, major U.S. brands	40	20–90
Brewed, imported brands	60	25–110
Instant	30	24–31
Iced	28	9–50
Some soft drinks, 12 ounces	35	20–40
Diet cola, 12 ounces	47	–
Cocoa beverage, 8 ounces	6	3–32
Chocolate milk beverage, 8 ounces	5	2–7
Milk chocolate, 1 ounce	6	1–15
Dark chocolate, semi-sweet, 1 ounce	20	5–35
Baker's chocolate, 1 ounce	26	1
Chocolate-flavored syrup, 1 ounce	4	1
Coffee-flavored frozen yogurt, 1 cup	85	1
Coffee ice cream, 1 cup	50	40–60
Coffee-flavored yogurt, 8 ounces	45	1

Source: International Food Information Council, Center for Science in the Public Interest

Cutting Back on Caffeine

If you're having trouble cutting back on caffeine, here are some tips to gradually wean yourself:

Mix half regular coffee with half decaffeinated.

Alternate a caffeinated beverage with a decaffeinated one throughout the day.

Drink caffeine-free soft drinks. Check the labels of clear and caramel-colored drinks for added caffeine.

Alcohol Matters

The effects of caffeine during pregnancy may be murky, but alcohol's consequences are crystal clear, and so is the recommendation for consumption: don't drink any alcohol if you are pregnant or trying to conceive.

Alcohol consumption deprives baby of the oxygen he needs, affecting the development of every one of his organs. Alcohol in pregnancy can cause physical and mental damage to your developing baby. At its worst, alcohol abuse causes fetal alcohol syndrome (FAS), a primary cause of mental retardation in the United States.

The consequences of regular, moderate alcohol consumption on a developing baby may be more subtle than FAS but just as devastating. As little as one to two drinks daily may cause miscarriage or low birth weight, which can put your baby at risk for developmental and health difficulties.

If you're concerned about the wine, beer, or mixed drinks you had before getting a positive pregnancy test, speak with your health care provider. If you are dependent on alcohol, seek professional help to stop drinking.

Is it OK...to drink decaffeinated coffee and tea, and herbal tea when pregnant?

Yes, within reason. Decaffeinated coffee and tea have nearly zero caffeine and are acceptable alternatives for women wishing to limit caffeine intake. Any type of coffee or tea interferes with nonheme iron absorption, so don't drink them with meals. Herbal teas have no caffeine, as long as they aren't mixed with regular tea. Herbal teas in pregnancy should be consumed with care, however. While most brand name herbal teas on supermarket shelves, such as apple-cinnamon, mint, or ginger tea, are safe for pregnancy, many other herbal teas, such as those sold in health food stores, may not be safe for pregnancy. For example, sassafras root is toxic to the liver, and most certainly dangerous to a developing baby. When in doubt, leave herbal tea out.

Lead: A Heavy Metal

If you live in a house built before 1986, there's a chance that your home plumbing contains lead, which can leach into your drinking water. Even the newer copper pipes that carry water into homes may have lead solder at their joints.

Lead builds up in your body over time, posing a serious health threat. Unborn babies are especially vulnerable to their mother's long-term lead exposure, which can increase the risk of miscarriage and stillbirths, and may result in long-term development problems, including brain damage and learning disability.

Lead sneaks into your life in other ways, too, some which you may not realize. For example, fluids allowed to sit in leaded crystal decanters become high in lead. Hot fluids, such as tea and coffee, can leach lead from lead-glazed mugs. Ceramic pottery with lead-containing glaze, usually imported, can add lead to your foods. And dwellings with chipping lead paint are high-risk places to live. Pregnant women should not be exposed to lead-paint removal.

If you're concerned about lead...

- ➤ Get your drinking water tested. Contact your local public health department to see if they can test it. Or call the Environmental Protection Agency (EPA) at (800) 426-4791 for a list of state-certified labs, and to get your questions about lead in drinking water answered.
- ➤ If you suspect lead in your pipes, let the cold water run for at least a minute before using the tap water for drinking or cooking purposes. Running the water flushes out the water that's been sitting in the pipes, which may have a large lead concentration.
- ➤ Opt for bottled water, which is typically lead-free.
- ➤ Avoid dwellings with chipping lead paint or where lead paint removal is taking place.

Chapter Five

An Eating Guide for Pregnancy

YOU'VE LEARNED ABOUT individual nutrients and their part in pregnancy. But you may be wondering how this translates to actual food choices for meals and snacks. The Food Guide Pyramid guides you to good nutrition at any stage of life. With a few minor adjustments, it works particularly well in pregnancy and breast-feeding.

Pyramid for Pregnancy

As you can see from the Food Guide Pyramid on the next page, a healthy eating plan in pregnancy is based on carbohydrates, including breads, grain products, pasta, fruits, and vegetables. High-protein foods such as dairy products, meat, poultry, eggs, and legumes are very important, too, and round out a healthful eating plan.

Eating well when expecting is all about balance. Your pregnancy food choices should reflect the variety of foods in each of the groups. Balancing high-fat fare with low-fat choices, and choosing a variety of foods in the right amounts, are the key to a healthy diet, pregnant or not. Read on for guidelines on how to put together a healthy pregnancy eating plan. To get you started, also refer to the sample menus in Appendix 2.

Serving Savvy

To use the Food Guide Pyramid for meal planning, you must first figure out how many servings you need daily from each food

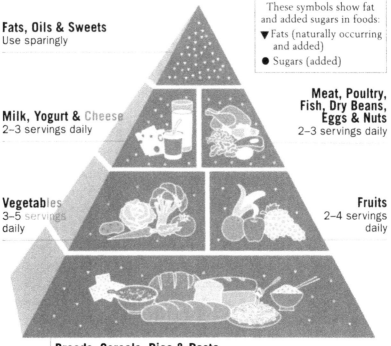

Fats, Oils & Sweets
Use sparingly

These symbols show fat and added sugars in foods:
▼ Fats (naturally occurring and added)
● Sugars (added)

Milk, Yogurt & Cheese
2–3 servings daily

Meat, Poultry, Fish, Dry Beans, Eggs & Nuts
2–3 servings daily

Vegetables
3–5 servings daily

Fruits
2–4 servings daily

Breads, Cereals, Rice & Pasta
6–11 servings daily

group. The following numbers figure in light to moderate activity. You may need more servings, especially if you're a teenager and if you're more active.

	Pregnant	**Breast-feeding**	**Non-pregnant**
Calories	about 2,500	about 2,700	1,600–1,800
Bread Group	9	10	6
Vegetable Group	4	4	3
Fruit Group	3	4	2
Milk Group*	3–4	3–4	2–3
Meat Group	2	2	2
	(6–7 oz. or equivalent)	(6–7 oz. or equivalent)	(5 oz. or equivalent)

*Teens need the highest number of servings from this group, if not more.

Serving sizes may be bigger, or smaller, than you think. What's important is that you meet the guidelines for minimum number of servings per day. Here are some examples from each food group, along with some best bets for nutrient-packed choices.

Breads, Cereal, Rice, and Pasta Group

A serving is:
- 1 slice bread (1 ounce)
- 1 ounce ready-to-eat cereal
- 1 ounce of hamburger or hot dog roll; pita bread; English muffin; or bagel
- 1 (6-inch) tortilla
- 1/2 cup cooked cereal or grain products, such as rice, pasta, or grits
- 3–4 small crackers
- 1 (4-inch diameter) pancake or waffle
- 3 tablespoons wheat germ
- 2 medium cookies

About this food group: The Bread group runs the gamut, from whole grain bread to cookies. This food group offers much in the way of nutrients, so make the most of your choices. For example, fiber, vitamins, and minerals, such as iron and folic acid found in fortified grains, are abundant in many of the choices you can make.

Best bets: Whole grain breads, cereals, and other grain products. Choose these more often, and go easy on cookies, cakes, and pastries.

Fruit Group

A serving is:
- 1 medium fruit
- 1/2 grapefruit, mango, or papaya
- 3/4 cup (6 ounces) juice
- 1/2 cup cut-up fruit, berries, or canned, cooked, or frozen fruit
- 1/4 cup dried fruit

About this food group: Fiber, folate, and phytochemicals (plant chemicals that fight off chronic illness) abound in the Fruit group, as do a host of other nutrients, including beta-carotene, and vitamin C.

Best bets: Pick the highest fiber fruits, and limit juice consumption (it's low in fiber) by mixing one serving with club soda or sparkling water. Try to include one source of vitamin C daily, such as an orange, half a grapefruit, or a kiwi. Satisfy your sweet tooth by using fruit as dessert—fresh or baked in a fruit crisp or cobbler. Or make yourself a Frozen Fruit Smoothie (see page 76).

Vegetable Group

A serving is:
1/2 cup cooked vegetables
1 cup raw, leafy vegetables
3/4 cup vegetable juice
1/2 cup chopped raw, nonleafy vegetables (such as carrots)
1 small baked potato or sweet potato

About this food group: A colorful array of vegetables with myriad nutrients, including fiber, folate, beta-carotene, vitamins C and E, and phytochemicals.

Best bets: Go for variety within this food group, and shoot for the highest fiber foods possible. Folate is found in dark green leafy vegetables; squash, carrots, and sweet potatoes supply beta-carotene; and tomatoes and green peppers help with iron absorption because they contain vitamin C. If you prefer vegetable juice, go for the reduced-sodium varieties.

Milk, Yogurt, and Cheese Group

A serving is:
1 cup (8 ounces) milk or yogurt, any type
1/2 cup evaporated milk
1/3 cup powdered milk

1 1/2 ounces natural cheese (mozzarella, Swiss, cheddar, Monterey Jack)

1/2 cup ricotta cheese

2 ounces processed cheese (American)

1 cup cottage cheese (equals 1/2 serving from this group)

1 cup frozen yogurt

1/2 cup ice cream (equals 1/3 serving from this group)

About this food group: Contains foods rich in calcium, and lots of other vitamins and minerals, as well as protein.

Best bets: Pick the lower fat choices more often, such as reduced-fat milk, cheese, yogurt, and frozen desserts, to get the biggest bang for your nutritional buck. For example, foods such as ice cream can count toward fulfilling your need from this food group, but at a much higher calorie "cost" than low-fat milk.

Meat, Poultry, Fish, Dry Beans, Eggs, and Nuts Group

A serving is:

2 to 3 ounces of cooked lean meat, poultry, or fish (about 4 ounces raw)

2 to 3 ounces lean sliced deli meat

For a total of 5 to 7 ounces daily

Counts as 1 ounce of meat, poultry, or fish:

1 egg

1/2 cup cooked lentils, peas, or dry beans

1/4 cup egg substitute

2 tablespoons peanut butter

1/3 cup nuts

4 ounces tofu, tempeh, or textured vegetable protein (TVP)

About this food group: What do nuts and meat have in common? Protein. Meat group selections are also rich in vitamin and minerals, and fiber in the case of legumes, nuts, and seeds. "Mainstream" and vegetarian food choices are represented here, with a varying fat content.

Best bets: Eating legumes, lean cuts of meat, skinless poultry, and seafood more often keeps calories in check and helps meet protein requirements.

Fats, Oils, and Sweets

The tip of the pyramid contains cream, butter, gravy, margarine, cream cheese, oils, salad dressings, sugars, fruit and soft drinks, jams and jellies, candy, sherbet, and gelatin desserts.

The Food Guide Pyramid advises using fats, oils, and sweets sparingly because they supply mostly calories, adding pleasure to eating with few nutrients. There are no designated portion sizes or limits because each person's "allowance" of fats, oils, and sweets varies depending on calorie needs.

Eating on the Run

We live in a grab-and-go society. If we didn't eat in our cars, at our desks, or in restaurants, some of us would hardly eat at all! When you're pregnant, it pays to slow down a bit to take stock of your eating habits and to better assess how to balance your eating style with your nutritional needs. Rushing around leaves you little time for eating well and for rest, both of which are essential to a healthy pregnancy.

Bolstering Breakfast

The facts are on the table. Breakfast eaters are better nourished. Think breakfast is boring? Or maybe you don't have the time or the appetite first thing in the morning, especially since you've been pregnant. Here are some enticements to eat one of the most important meals of the day. You can even take some of these suggestions and use them as snacks.

➤ Stock your home or office with high-fiber, low-fat cereal, milk, and fresh or dried fruit. Trade in your rushed morning routine for a 5-minute sit-down meal of 1 cup of cereal, 8 ounces of milk, and a serving of fruit.

➤ Before you leave the house, or the night before, construct a graham cracker sandwich for breakfast. Take two graham crackers, smear with peanut butter, and add a layer of sliced banana. Top it off with a glass of milk.

➤ Pick up a container of yogurt, a small bagel or whole grain roll, and a carton of juice on your way to work, or in the company cafeteria.

A break from tradition...

➤ Start with a tortilla. Layer with two slices of turkey breast and one slice cheese. Roll up. Eat with a piece of fruit.

➤ Microwave leftover pizza and eat in the car. Add a carton of juice when you get to your destination.

➤ Try a hot soft pretzel, piece of fresh fruit, and carton of milk.

When you have a few minutes at home...

➤ Swirl chunky applesauce and raisins into hot oatmeal. Enjoy with 8 ounces of milk.

➤ Microwave a frozen pancake (or make from scratch). Spread with 2 tablespoons peanut butter and top with raisins. Roll it up crepe-style.

➤ For a perfect parfait: Layer yogurt, fresh fruit, and your favorite cereal.

Make it and go...

➤ Split a bagel, and spread each half with hummus or peanut butter. Bring along 8 ounces juice or milk.

➤ Boil some eggs. Peel one before work and wrap in a plastic bag. Eat it on your way to work, along with a bagel and fruit.

➤ Whip up a Frozen Fruit Smoothie (see page 76) and pour into an insulated cup to sip on the go.

Lunch on the Fly

Lunch should provide about a third of your daily nutrient requirements. Skipping or skimping on lunch can make it difficult to meet your needs. Here are some ways to make it count.

....

Building a Better Salad

Regardless of where you build your salad, here are ways to construct a nutritious salad.

Foundation—Dark, leafy greens, such as spinach or romaine.

First level—Plain vegetables. Add an array of color: broccoli, carrots, tomatoes, green and red bell pepper, and beets, for example.

Second story—Protein sources, including beans, cheese, egg, tofu, plain tuna, and turkey breast.

Trimmings—Reduced-fat salad dressing.

Addition—2 ounces bread, such as 2 slices whole wheat or a medium roll.

Sandwich Savvy

Restaurant food can be higher in calories, fat, and sodium than homemade. Sandwiches are no exception. For example, a typical tuna fish sandwich can contain more than 700 calories and 43 grams of fat! Many restaurant wrap sandwiches register at least 1,000 milligrams of sodium, and some contain upwards of 3,500 milligrams. They're not all bad, however: A commercially-prepared turkey with mustard weighs in around 370 calories.

If you're a regular sandwich buyer, limit excess calories by ordering turkey or roast beef on whole grain bread; ask for mustard instead of mayonnaise; and request reduced-fat cheese. Even better, split large sandwiches with a friend, or save half for later.

Common sense tells you it may be cheaper and healthier to prepare sandwiches at home. It takes just a few minutes of your time to prepare a sandwich to take with you. Here are some recipes for sandwiches that will save you money and calories in the long run. Experiment with different whole grain breads, including pita, and try making your own wrap sandwiches with a tortilla.

Beef, Turkey, or Ham: 2 to 3 ounces meat (2 to 3 medium slices); or 2 ounces meat and 1 ounce cheese. Add mustard or reduced-fat mayonnaise, lettuce, and tomato. Place fillings in the center of a flour tortilla and roll it up.

Chicken, Egg, or Tuna Salad: Mix 2 to 3 ounces tuna fish, chicken, or 2 hard-cooked eggs with 2 to 3 teaspoons reduced-fat mayonnaise. Add celery or onion to the tuna, chicken, or egg salad, or for a change, add chopped grapes to chicken salad. Spread on a whole-grain roll. Add a few leaves of romaine lettuce and tomato.

Vegetarian: Combine chopped vegetables with such legumes as 1/4 cup garbanzos or another favorite bean, and add 1 to 2 ounces cheese, such as feta. Toss mixture with 1 to 2 teaspoons reduced-fat salad dressing. Stuff into a large whole-wheat pita pocket half.

Simplifying Supper

It's the end of the day. You may be tired and may not feel like spending time to prepare a big meal. Supper doesn't have to be fancy or elaborate to be nutritious and satisfying. Go for meals that contain foods from at least three of the five food groups. Here are ideas for simplifying supper:

➤ Shop regularly.

➤ Make food ahead. For example, prepare a double batch of beef stew, or roast a chicken or turkey on the weekends. Add a grain and a vegetable and you've got a meal!

➤ Serve breakfast foods for dinner. Too tired to cook, or even think about eating? Turn the day on its ear. Why not have scrambled eggs, toast, and fruit for supper? Or try French toast with fruit, or cereal, milk, and fruit.

➤ Capitalize on convenience foods. Prepackaged vegetables like baby carrots, salad greens, and cherry tomatoes can be the basis of a healthy main meal salad, or side vegetable. For instance, add chopped, leftover chicken to pasta sauce from a jar for a quick meal. Top it off with fruit and bread.

➤ Soup and a sandwich. Have on hand reduced-sodium soups, such as lentil, and pair up with a simple sandwich, such as grilled cheese or tuna fish. Add a salad or piece of fruit.

➤ Remember to enjoy a glass of milk with your meal.

Snacking

Snacks are small meals often mistakenly portrayed as appetite wreckers and the reason for weight gain. But snacking wisely is a healthy habit, especially when pregnant, because snacks can fill in nutrient gaps and keep energy levels high and nausea at bay. Make sure your snacks figure into your total allotment of food group servings so they don't end up promoting excessive weight gain.

Here are some healthy snacks to have on hand:

➤ Bagels
➤ Dried fruit
➤ Fresh fruit
➤ Juice
➤ Low-fat crackers, such as soda crackers, and graham crackers
➤ Raw vegetables and yogurt-based dip or hummus
➤ Ready-to-eat cereal
➤ Yogurt
➤ Fig bars
➤ Pretzels
➤ Frozen yogurt
➤ Cottage cheese

Chapter Six

An Active
Pregnancy

YOU MAY HAVE worked out before conceiving. The good news is that you can continue with physical activity right up until delivery, if you're willing and able. Why be active when pregnant? Regular physical activity increases energy, maintains muscle tone, endurance, and strength, reduces stress, and helps you sleep better. It may also help to prevent varicose veins. Exercising moms-to-be don't necessarily have less painful or shorter deliveries. But moderate physical activity during pregnancy may provide the stamina to withstand a long labor, should you have one.

Chances are you can continue with the same exercise routine—with a few modifications and exceptions. For example, any activity that involves pressure changes (which could deprive the baby of oxygen) or falls, such as sky diving, scuba diving, downhill skiing, water skiing, and horseback riding, are not advised during pregnancy. You may also want to trade peddling your bike in traffic for riding on a bike trail, to be safer. If you do not exercise regularly, but want to start during pregnancy, ask your health care provider first.

Physical Activity Tips

The American College of Obstetricians and Gynecologists (ACOG) has developed exercise guidelines for pregnancy. If you don't have a high-risk pregnancy, exercising at least three times weekly is beneficial. Always consult your doctor before working out when expecting. Here are some ACOG exercising do's and don'ts:

> **Don't** exercise while lying down (for example, sit-ups) after the first trimester.

> **Do** lower your exercise intensity, and don't exercise to exhaustion (especially during the last trimester, when pregnancy is putting a strain on your circulatory system).

> **Do** make sure you're getting enough calories to ensure adequate weight gain.

> **Don't** do deep stretching or jerky, bouncy motions, such as jumping, or rapidly changing directions.

> **Do** stop activity immediately if you feel any pain or discomfort.

> **Do** gradually resume your workouts after giving birth, starting 4 to 6 weeks after delivery, as you are able, and after your health care provider gives you the go-ahead.

> **Don't** get overheated.

Special Concerns

Pregnant women often comment on how warm they feel. Your body produces more heat during pregnancy because your metabolism is revved up. The same thing happens when you exercise; working muscles produce heat that your body must get rid of.

When you're pregnant, it's important to keep your core body temperature within a normal range, around 98.6 degrees Fahrenheit. When you do not release body heat, your core temperature can rise to dangerous levels, possibly compromising your baby's brain development. Inadequate fluid intake and exercising in a warm environment, such as a poorly ventilated, crowded aerobics room or gym, or hot, humid weather can result in overheating. High body temperature in pregnant women can also be caused by prolonged fever and hot tub use.

Keep coolest by exercising in well-ventilated, or cool conditions. And get enough fluid. Drink at least 8 ounces of water before exercise; sip another 8 ounces for every 15 to 20 minutes of exercise; and drink another 8 to 16 ounces after working out, thirsty or not. That may sound like a lot of fluid, but you need it.

You'll know you're getting enough fluid when you check your urine. If urine is plentiful and clear, you have a normal water balance. When it is dark and scanty, you need to drink more.

••

Figuring Fluid

Your fluid needs for a half-hour walk or bike ride in a cool gym:

Before exercise begins: At least 8 ounces water

During exercise: 16 ounces water

After exercise: At least 8 ounces water

Total: At least 32 ounces water

••

Chapter Seven

Managing the Discomforts of Pregnancy

MANY OF THE discomforts of pregnancy relate to what you eat, and range from occasional nausea to more serious conditions, such as elevated blood pressure. Find out why you might be experiencing certain problems and use the following suggestions to prevent or minimize the discomforts that may accompany your pregnancy. Read about some more serious health concerns related to nutrition in Chapter 8. Of course, you'll also want to discuss any discomforts or concerns with your health care provider.

Morning Sickness

What it is: "Morning sickness" runs the gamut. Some women have mild nausea, while others experience persistent vomiting that puts them at risk for dehydration and weight loss. "Morning sickness" is a misnomer because it can occur at any time of the day. It often subsides after the first trimester, but some women experience nausea throughout their pregnancy.

Why it happens: No one is exactly sure, but morning sickness is probably due to the many changes occurring in your body, including a rise in hormone levels.

What to do about it: Let your health care provider know if you vomit two or more times daily. But, if morning sickness is more of an irritation than a health threat, try these tips:

➤ Avoid offensive smells, since they can trigger nausea.

- Figure out what foods or beverages ease your nausea, and eat them. Even if they are soda and snack chips, they are better than nothing at all.
- Keep your bedroom window cracked at least one to two inches when sleeping, provided noise or safety are not an issue. Stale bedroom air can set off nausea.
- Get enough fluids. If you're nauseated, try to drink liquids that you can tolerate to help keep you hydrated. When you vomit, fluid loss occurs, and fluids must be replaced. If vomiting is severe and prolonged, hospitalization may be required to treat dehydration.
- Don't allow yourself to get too hungry. Keeping food in your stomach with small snacks seems to keep nausea at bay for many women.

Heartburn

What it is: Heartburn is another misnomer: it has nothing to do with your heart and everything to do with your stomach and esophagus. That irritation and sour taste in your mouth comes from highly acidic stomach juices spilling into your esophagus.

Why it happens: In the beginning of pregnancy, heartburn is due to hormonal changes that slow the movement of food through the digestive tract. As your pregnancy progresses, the baby's increasing size puts pressure on your internal organs, crowding the stomach and causing stomach acid to back up into the esophagus.

What to do: One or more of these strategies may ease your heartburn symptoms.
- Don't lay down right after eating since this can aggravate heartburn.
- Sleep with your head slightly elevated to decrease acid back up.
- Try eating frequent, small meals, especially in the third trimester.
- Avoid known irritants, including caffeine, chocolate, and highly-seasoned foods, and any other food that bothers you.
- Ask your health care provider about taking antacids.

Constipation

What it is: Infrequent stools or hard, dry stools.

Why it happens: Pregnancy slows down the movement of food through your digestive tract. Additionally, constipation is a side effect of taking supplemental iron, either from a prenatal multi-vitamin and mineral supplement or a separate iron supplement. Inadequate fiber, fluid, and physical exercise can aggravate constipation, too.

What to do:
- Keep taking prescribed supplements.
- Include high fiber foods in your daily food choices. Aim for 20 to 35 grams of fiber daily (see "Focus on Fiber" on page 7.)
- Drink at least 64 ounces (8 cups) of caffeine-free fluids daily to enhance fiber's laxative effects.
- Get regular physical activity, which stimulates your digestive tract, to promote regular bowel movements.
- If constipation persists, ask your health care provider if you can divide your iron dose during the day or take the supplement with food.

Hemorrhoids

What they are: Dilated, engorged veins surrounding the rectum. They cause itching and sometimes, severe pain.

Why they happen: May occur with straining to move your bowels due to constipation, or with pushing during childbirth.

What to do:
- Prevent constipation by following the tips above.
- Include plenty of fiber and fluids to keep your stools soft.
- If you have a severe case, ask your health care provider about treatment.

Swelling

What it is: Extra water held in and around your cells.

Why it happens: Your blood volume expands in pregnancy, and so does the amount of water cells hold. Some swelling is normal, and some is not (see Pre-eclampsia in Chapter 8).

What to do:

> ➤ It may sound funny, but drink more water.
> ➤ Don't restrict your sodium intake.
> ➤ Elevate your feet whenever possible. Avoid standing for long periods.
> ➤ Consult your health care provider if swelling seems excessive.

Food Aversions

What they are: Quite suddenly, you can't stand the sight or smell of a certain food. It may even be a food that you once loved and ate regularly.

Why they happen: No one knows. And a food aversion may disappear as quickly as it came on.

What to do:

> ➤ Don't be concerned, unless you can't stomach an entire food group.
> ➤ If possible, leave the cooking to someone else and stay away from food preparation areas.
> ➤ Try eating foods cold or at room temperature since the aroma will be minimized.
> ➤ Consult a registered dietitian for a healthy food plan if you find that you're not eating a variety of foods.

Is it OK...to take laxatives if you're constipated?

Possibly. But before you rely on medication to relieve constipation, give the power of food a fair chance. Try to get at least 20 grams of fiber daily (see "Focus on Fiber," page 7) and at least eight glasses of caffeine-free beverages daily to fight constipation. Regular physical activity helps, too. If those tricks don't work, ask your doctor about laxatives. Never take any medication without first consulting a licensed health care professional who knows you're pregnant.

Chapter Eight

Special Concerns During Pregnancy

IF YOU'RE LIKE most pregnant women, you probably have many concerns related to your pregnancy. This chapter looks at several different health concerns that may or may not pertain to you. All pregnant women should be concerned about keeping food safe—be sure to read the tips for preventing foodborne illness. If you follow a vegetarian eating style, you'll want to read about nutrients that may be lacking in vegetarian diets. Lastly, read about more serious health concerns and how to prevent and treat them.

Food Safety

Safe food is always important, but it's paramount in pregnancy. It's riskier for pregnant women to have foodborne illness because the vomiting and diarrhea that often occur with foodborne illness can result in dehydration, nutrient loss, and fluid imbalance. Keep foodborne illness at bay with these food safety rules.

➤ Wash your hands with warm soapy water for at least 20 seconds before handling food and between tasks involving raw meat, poultry, and fish.

➤ Rinse fruits and vegetables well before eating. Remove outer leaves of greens before eating or cooking.

➤ Keep hot foods hot (140 degrees F and above) and cold foods cold (maximum of 40 degrees F). Do not allow cooked food containing meat, poultry, fish, eggs, or dairy products to sit at room temperature for more than 2 hours.

➤ Never consume raw or undercooked meat, poultry, seafood, or eggs. In addition, steer clear of soft cheeses, including Brie, feta, blue cheese, and Camembert, and never drink unpasteurized juice and milk. For example, avoid Caesar salad dressing unless it's made with pasteurized eggs, as well as eggnog made with raw eggs. (Most commercial eggnogs are pasteurized.) And forego foods like apple cider from roadside stands, unless you know it's been pasteurized.

➤ Wash and rinse all surfaces and utensils that come in contact with raw meat, fish, or poultry.

➤ Cook meat, poultry, and seafood thoroughly. Make sure ground meat or poultry, pork, and ham is cooked to at least 160 degrees F; steaks, roasts, and fish to at least 145 degrees F; and poultry parts (breasts, thighs, and wings) to at least 170 degrees F before eating.

➤ Change sponges, dishcloths, and dishrags frequently.

➤ When in doubt, toss food out. If you suspect food has gone bad or has not been handled properly, it's best to be safe and throw it out. Don't rely on your nose for detecting whether a food is safe to eat. Food that contains foodborne illness-causing bacteria will not necessarily smell or look spoiled.

➤ Buy only properly-handled food. For example, never purchase unrefrigerated eggs, meat, or seafood.

➤ Don't thaw foods on the countertop.

➤ Set your refrigerator at 35 to 40 degrees F, and make sure it stays in this range.

Flu or Foodborne Illness?

You've been feeling flu-like for hours. If the symptoms don't go away within 24 to 48 hours, you could have something more serious, such as foodborne illness. Be safe and let your health care provider know. Call your health care provider immediately when one or more of the following symptoms occur:

You vomit, or have diarrhea, more than two times a day,

Your diarrhea is bloody,

You have all of these symptoms simultaneously: stiff neck, severe headache, and fever,

Your symptoms last for more than three days.

The Vegetarian Mom-to-Be

If you've chosen vegetarianism as your eating style and you include dairy products and eggs (also known as lacto-ovo vegetarianism), then you'll have few nutritional hurdles during pregnancy, since eating adequate amounts of dairy products and eggs along with a well-balanced diet will provide the pregnancy nutrition you need. On the other hand, vegan moms-to-be, who exclude all animal products, have to be more vigilant about getting the nutrients they need for a healthy pregnancy.

Whatever type of vegetarianism you favor, it pays to see a registered dietitian about your eating choices during pregnancy. Here are a few nutrients that may be at issue in vegetarian pregnancy diets. Refer to Appendixes 1 and 2 for suggested serving amounts and sample menus for lacto-ovo vegetarian diets.

Protein

Since protein is found in both animal and plant foods, vegetarians who eat enough dairy products, eggs, or plant-based foods typically have little trouble getting the protein they need in pregnancy. Gone are the days when vegans worried about combining plant foods to achieve the right protein mix for good health. As long as you eat a wide variety of plant foods, including whole grains, cereals, and legumes, you can get the protein that you and your baby need.

Special Concerns During Pregnancy

Calcium and Vitamin D

Pregnant women require 1,000 milligrams of calcium daily. Calcium is found in both animal and plant foods. The calcium in foods such as milk, cheese, and yogurt is particularly well-absorbed by the body. Milk is an especially beneficial source of calcium because it also contains vitamin D, which boosts calcium absorption and deposition in your bones and in your developing baby's.

You can satisfy your daily calcium requirement with at least three to four servings from the Milk, Yogurt, and Cheese group. See Chapter 5 for serving size guidelines. As an added benefit, dairy products are also good sources of protein.

If you don't eat dairy, concentrate on including calcium-rich plant foods to get the 1,000 daily milligrams of calcium you need when expecting. See Calcium Countdown on page 20 for the calcium content of some plant foods.

Few foods contain vitamin D naturally. Several foods are fortified with the vitamin, though, including most milk products, some ready-to-eat cereals, and fortified soy milk. In addition, your body can make its own vitamin D by the action of sunlight on the skin. (Read more about vitamin D on page 16.) Some vegans may require supplemental vitamin D, but don't take any supplement without first asking a registered dietitian or your health care provider.

Iron

Many women take a prescribed prenatal vitamin and mineral supplement during pregnancy that includes iron to meet increased needs and prevent iron-deficiency anemia. As a vegetarian mom-to-be, it is difficult to meet your increased iron needs if you don't include animal products, especially meat. If you follow a vegetarian eating style, talk to your health care provider about taking an iron supplement. You should also try to include plant sources of iron as well as iron-fortified foods. And make an effort to include a source of vitamin C with your iron-containing foods to enhance absorption of iron. See page 24 for more information on iron sources.

Vitamin B$_{12}$

Since vitamin B$_{12}$ is found primarily in animal foods, pregnant vegans should be sure their diets contain plant-based food sources of vitamin B$_{12}$ to help prevent a form of anemia. Fortified breakfast cereals provide vitamin B$_{12}$, as do fortified soy milks and some other nondairy milks. Nutritional yeast, such as Red Star Vegetarian Support Formula, supplies vitamin B$_{12}$, while brewer's yeast does not.

Zinc

Zinc is needed for cell growth and repair, as well as energy production. Zinc is found in many animal foods, including milk, meat, cheese, yogurt, and eggs, so if you eat enough of these foods, chances are you'll get all the zinc you need.

If you avoid all animal foods, concentrate on eating zinc-containing plant foods, such as whole wheat bread; whole grains, such as bran flakes and wheat germ; legumes and peas; tofu; seeds; and nuts. Do not take a zinc supplement without first discussing it with your health care provider or dietitian.

Special Health Conditions During Pregnancy

Iron-Deficiency Anemia

What it is: A blood disorder characterized by chronic fatigue, irritability, and lack of concentration.

Why it happens: The demand for iron increases beginning in the second trimester. Pregnant women with deficient iron reserves and an iron-poor diet may not make sufficient hemoglobin, the part of the red blood cell that transports oxygen. The baby is not likely to suffer from iron-deficiency anemia, but the effects on mom can be serious.

What to do:
- ➤ Take all prescribed iron supplements.
- ➤ Get enough iron from foods (see "Iron Clad Foods" on page 24.)
- ➤ To maximize iron absorption from plant foods, eat plant foods with vitamin C-containing foods or an animal source of iron.

Pre-eclampsia

What it is: Pre-eclampsia is marked by fluid retention in the hands and face, sudden weight gain, elevated blood pressure, protein in the urine, and decreased blood flow to the baby.

Why it happens: Pre-eclampsia may be associated with inadequate nutrient intake, but no one knows for sure why it occurs. For example, adequate protein and minerals promote proper fluid balance, blood volume, and tissue growth. And for protein to do its job, you also must get adequate calories. Inadequate nutrition before and during pregnancy can increase pre-eclampsia risk.

What to do:
- ➤ To help reduce chances of pre-eclampsia, eat a well-balanced diet before conception and during pregnancy.
- ➤ Follow your health care provider's advice.

Gestational Diabetes

What it is: A form of diabetes that affects about 4 percent of pregnant American women, according to the American Diabetes Association. Gestational diabetes usually appears later in pregnancy and is more common in overweight women with a family history of the disease. Diabetes in pregnancy increases risk for high blood pressure, and makes for bigger babies that are more difficult to deliver and may have breathing problems.

Why it happens: Pregnancy creates extra demands on your pancreas, which produces insulin to help keep blood glucose levels normal. If the pancreas can't keep up, the concentration of glucose is chronically above normal in your blood, the condition known as diabetes. Gestational diabetes often disappears after childbirth but may result in diabetes later in life.

What to do:
- ➤ Keep blood glucose levels as normal as possible.
- ➤ See a registered dietitian for help to create a well-balanced meal plan.
- ➤ Follow your health care provider's or endocrinologist's (diabetes specialist) advice to the letter about how to best treat your gestational diabetes.

Chapter Nine

Postpartum Nutrition

YOU'VE DELIVERED YOUR bundle of joy, and now you want your figure back. How long will it take to shed baby weight? The good news first: you drop a significant portion of what you gained in pregnancy during the first few weeks after delivery. The not-so-great news: losing the remaining weight and getting back muscle tone can take up to a year.

A year? That's right, but don't fret. Life is hectic after baby comes. Whether or not you are nursing, you should wait at least 6 weeks post-delivery before beginning a weight-loss regimen that restricts calories and includes physical activity. You need all the energy you can get—to recover from giving birth, deal with the needs of an infant, help manage a household, and possibly return to work—all on less sleep. So, cut yourself some slack. You will get your body back. For now, enjoy your little one, eat healthily, and try to fit in moderate physical activity when you can.

Weighing In on Weight Control

If You're Breast-Feeding

Breast-feeding does not magically melt away pounds, but it can help. Milk production alone requires about 800 calories daily. Stored body fat from pregnancy kicks in about 300 calories a day for producing milk and your diet should contribute the rest. That means you need to eat an extra 500 calories to supply the necessary nursing energy. That's 200 more calories than you needed during pregnancy!

How many calories are right for you? On average, most women need about 2,700 calories a day when nursing. In your quest for fitness, you may be tempted to eat less. Health professionals warn that eating fewer than 1,800 calories a day may decrease milk production and sap the energy that you need to feed and care for an infant.

Add moderate physical activity, such as walking or following an exercise video, only when your doctor gives you the go ahead. The benefits of taking baby for regular walks are twofold: you and baby get fresh air while seeing the sights; and physical activity fosters weight loss without drastically cutting calories. If it's tough to get outside, invest in a few exercise videotapes, and let baby watch as you work out, or exercise when baby sleeps. If you find yourself losing more than about 4 pounds a month after cutting calories and adding exercise, add back some calories.

When you're breast-feeding, what you eat affects your baby's health and how quickly you recover from giving birth. For example, you can maximize the vitamin content of your breast milk by eating the healthiest diet possible. Same goes for bolstering your iron stores. It can take months to make up for the iron you lost in blood during childbirth. To replenish nutrient stores, focus on healthy eating and ask your health care provider whether you should continue taking prescribed prenatal supplements. Refer to Chapter 5 for healthy eating guidelines based on the Food Guide Pyramid. Since you are capable of getting pregnant when nursing, the same guidelines apply about getting adequate folate (see Folate on page 17).

Fluids are central to breast milk production. To get enough, sip on caffeine-free beverages throughout the day, and try to drink 8 ounces of water each time you sit down to nurse your baby. For the most part, limit alcohol and caffeine. They make their way into your milk and they cause water loss.

If You Don't Breast-Feed

Many of the same principles of weight loss apply even when you don't breast-feed. For example, you need your strength, so put off restricting calories for at least six weeks. And when you begin your weight control regimen, make sure you eat a variety of foods from all of the food groups to ensure adequate nutrients for replenishing your body's stores. When you're ready to begin physical activity, do so gradually.

How many calories for weight loss? Most women do well by consuming at least 1,600 to 1,800 calories a day along with light activity to help drop the weight and keep it off. That calorie level may sound high, especially to repeat dieters, who often eat 1,200 calories daily, or less. But eating at least a 1,600-calorie diet is far more reasonable, because it gives you room to include the minimum number of servings from all five food groups, which will boost your energy level and promote good health. And 1,600 calories a day is much easier to stick with in the long run because you're less likely to feel deprived at this calorie level.

Use the Food Guide Pyramid and the Nutrition Facts panel on food labels to help meet your calorie and nutrient goals. See Chapter 5 for meal planning help.

••

Move It and Lose It

You may not make it to the gym as often as you did before baby came along, but it probably feels like you are more active. The daily chores involved with taking care of an infant and running a household may burn more calories than you think, so don't dismiss "informal" workouts.

Burn 150 calories by:

Washing windows and floors for 45 to 60 minutes
Gardening for 30 to 45 minutes
Pushing a stroller 1 1/2 miles in 30 minutes
Raking leaves for 30 minutes
Walking two miles in 30 minutes
Shoveling snow for 15 minutes
Walking up stairs for 15 minutes

Source: Physical Activity and Health: A Report of the Surgeon General, Centers for Disease Control and Prevention, 1996.

••

Weight Loss Readiness

If you're thinking about starting a weight control program to drop post-baby pounds—either on your own or through a commercial program—ask yourself the following questions:

➤ Are you ready to work on losing the weight, and keeping it off? You're probably busy, and weight loss demands commitment. Keep in mind that commercial weight control programs often demand money up front. You'll want to assess whether you need the support and motivation from a commercial program before plunking down your money.

➤ Does the program offer an eating plan for nursing women, and does it take into account your individual nutrient needs?

➤ Does the program encourage a safe, personalized physical activity program?

➤ What promises does the program make about rate of weight loss? A safe and realistic rate of weight loss is about 1 to 2 pounds weekly, about 1 pound a week if you're nursing.

➤ What is the format? Group settings foster peer support, while one-to-one counseling speaks directly to your nutritional needs. Self-directed plans also work well for some women. Consider which is best for you.

➤ Does the eating plan exclude any of the five food groups? If it does, drop it like a hot potato. It's unhealthy and especially dangerous for breast-feeding women.

➤ Will the program help you make lasting eating changes? Check out the philosophy and rationale. See if the program fosters long term behavior changes.

➤ For commercial programs, find out about fees—hidden and otherwise. Determine whether you'll be required to buy special foods and supplements, and figure that into a monthly or weekly cost so you'll know your total cost up front.

Is it OK...to start physical activity soon after delivery?

Give it at least 4 to 6 weeks before you begin including regular physical activity again, says the American College of Obstetricians and Gynecologists. When you do take on physical activity, keep it gentle, and listen to your body. Activity has many benefits, including faster and more lasting weight loss; improved muscle tone and self-esteem; decreased stress; and increased energy. Be sure to get your health care provider's OK before you resume any exercise after delivery.

Before Your Next Baby

Contemplating another pregnancy? It's never too early to lay the groundwork for conception. You'll want to bolster your nutrient reserves to give your next child the brightest of beginnings. Here's your preconception checklist.

➤ Consider waiting at least a year to conceive. Pregnancy and nursing are taxing on your body. Bearing children in quick succession puts added strain on your nutrient stores, such as calcium and iron, and on your energy level, especially if you're nursing.

➤ Don't severely restrict calories in an attempt to lose weight from your first pregnancy. Very low calorie diets are notoriously low in important pregnancy nutrients, including calcium, iron, and folate.

➤ If you are capable of becoming pregnant, be sure to include 400 micrograms of folate every day, either through food or dietary supplements. Health professionals estimate that 50 percent of pregnancies are unplanned. Remember that you need to get enough folate early in pregnancy—when you may not even know you're pregnant. (Read more about folate on page 17.)

➤ Don't smoke, drink, or take illicit drugs.

➤ Ask your doctor about over-the-counter medications you use, or are planning to take.

➤ Schedule time for rest and relaxation—easier said than done with a small child or two around the house, but no less important for good health.

Your Daily Food Checklist

WONDERING IF YOU'RE eating enough of the right foods? Keep tabs with this handy record. Copy and carry it with you to tally daily food choices.

Breads, Cereal, Rice, and Pasta Group

A serving is:
  1 slice bread (1 ounce)
  1 ounce ready-to-eat cereal
  1/2 of hamburger or hot dog roll; pita bread; English
    muffin; or bagel
  1 (6-inch) tortilla
  1/2 cup cooked cereal, pasta or grain, such as rice or grits
  3–4 small crackers
  1 (4-inch diameter) pancake or waffle
  3 tablespoons wheat germ
  2 medium cookies

Minimum Goals:
Pregnancy: 9 servings
Breast-feeding: 10 servings
Lacto-ovovegetarian Pregnancy and Breastfeeding: 9 servings
Non-Pregnant: 6 servings

Your total for the day: _____

Fruit Group

A serving is:
- 1 medium fruit
- 1/2 grapefruit, mango, or papaya
- 3/4 cup (6 ounces) juice
- 1/2 cup cut-up fruit, berries, or canned, cooked or frozen fruit
- 1/4 cup dried fruit

Minimum Goals:
Pregnancy: 3 servings
Breast-feeding: 4 servings
Lacto-ovovegetarian Pregnancy and Breast-feeding: 4 servings
Non-pregnant: 2 servings

Your total for the day: _____

Vegetable Group

A serving is:
- 1/2 cup cooked vegetables
- 1 cup raw, leafy vegetables
- 3/4 cup vegetable juice
- 1/2 cup chopped raw, nonleafy vegetables (such as carrots)
- 1 small baked potato or sweet potato

Minimum Goals:
Pregnancy and Breast-feeding: 4 servings
Lacto-ovovegetarian Pregnancy and Breast-feeding: 4 servings
Non-pregnant: 3 servings

Your total for the day: _____

Milk, Yogurt, and Cheese Group

A serving is:
- 1 cup (8 ounces) of milk or yogurt, any type
- 1/2 cup evaporated milk
- 1/3 cup powdered milk

1 1/2 ounces natural cheese (mozzarella, Swiss, cheddar,
   Monterey Jack)
1/2 cup ricotta cheese
2 ounces processed cheese (American)
1 cup cottage cheese (count as 1/2 serving)
1 cup frozen yogurt
1/2 cup ice cream (count as 1/3 serving)

Minimum Goals:
Pregnancy and Breast-feeding: 3 servings
Lacto-ovovegetarian Pregnancy and Breast-feeding: 4 servings (or as
many as 9 if dairy foods are a primary protein source)
Pregnant teenager: 4 servings
Non-pregnant: 2 servings

Your total for the day: _____

Meat, Poultry, Fish, Dry Beans, Eggs, and Nuts Group

A serving is:
2 to 3 ounces of cooked lean meat, poultry, or fish (about
   4 ounces raw)
2 to 3 ounces lean sliced deli meat
(for a total of 5 to 7 ounces daily)

Count as 1 ounce of meat, poultry or fish:
1 egg
1/2 cup cooked lentils, peas, or dry beans
1/4 cup egg substitute
2 tablespoons peanut butter
1/3 cup nuts
4 ounces tofu, tempeh, or textured vegetable protein
   (TVP)

Minimum Goals:
Pregnancy and Breast-feeding: 6 ounces or equivalents
Lacto-ovovegetarian Pregnancy and Breast-feeding: 6 ounces or
equivalents
Non-pregnant: 5 ounces or equivalents

Your total for the day: _____

Your Daily Food Checklist

Fats, Oils, and Sweets

There's no need to avoid the items in this group, like butter, margarine, salad dressing, and sweets, but treat these as extras and use them sparingly.

Sample Daily Meal Plans

THESE MEAL PLANS are examples of how to use the Food Guide Pyramid to plan a diet for pregnancy and breast-feeding. Each menu provides about 2,400 to 2,800 calories; the lower calorie figures reflect the use of low-calorie and low-fat products, such as fat-free milk, reduced-fat or fat-free salad dressings, and light margarine.

Day One

Breakfast
1 scrambled egg
2 pieces toast
1 teaspoon butter or margarine
1 medium orange
1 cup (8 ounces) milk

Snack
1/2 cup (4 ounces) juice

Lunch
2 ounces turkey
2 slices whole grain bread
1 slice reduced-fat cheddar
  cheese (1 1/2 ounces)
2 teaspoons reduced-fat mayonnaise or mustard
1 ounce pretzels
1 medium apple
1 cup (8 ounces) milk

Snack
4 graham cracker squares

Dinner
2 Beef Wraps (see Recipes)
1 cup cooked broccoli or carrots
1 teaspoon butter or margarine
1 cup (8 ounces) milk
1 piece or 1/2 cup chopped fresh
  fruit

Snack
Decaffeinated tea
Bread Pudding (see Recipes)

Day Two

Breakfast
1 cup high-fiber cereal
1 cup (8 ounces) milk
1 medium banana

Snack
1 piece fresh fruit or
1/4 cup dried fruit

Lunch
Chef's salad:
    2 cups salad greens
    1 cup raw sliced vegetables
    2 ounces tuna fish
    1 ounce Swiss cheese
    2 tablespoons salad dressing
1 large whole grain roll
    (2 ounces)
1 cup (8 ounces) milk
1 piece or 1/2 cup chopped fresh
    fruit

Snack
Bran and Molasses Muffin (see
    Recipes)

Dinner
Chicken and Apples, 1 serving
    (see Recipes)
1 1/2 cups cooked noodles
2 teaspoons butter or margarine
1 cup steamed broccoli
1 cup (8 ounces) milk

Snack
6 graham cracker squares
1 cup (8 ounces) milk

Day Three

Breakfast
Frozen Fruit Smoothie (see
    Recipes)

Snack
1/2 bagel (1 ounce)
2 teaspoons peanut butter

Lunch
Roast beef sandwich:
    2 ounces roast beef
    2 slices whole grain bread
    1 tablespoon reduced-fat may-
        onnaise or mustard
    lettuce and tomato
Small salad:
    1 cup greens
    1/2 cup raw vegetables, your
        choice
    1 tablespoon low-fat dressing
1 cup (8 ounces) milk
Fresh fruit, your choice

Snack
Healthy Hummus, 1/4 cup (see
    Recipes)
1/2 cup raw vegetables

Dinner
Zucchini Frittata, 1 serving (see
    Recipes)
1 1/2 cups cooked rice
1–2 teaspoons butter or mar-
    garine
1 cup steamed green beans
1 cup (8 ounces) milk
Fresh fruit, your choice

Snack
6 cups popped popcorn

Lacto-ovovegetarian Meal Plans

Day One

Breakfast
1 scrambled egg
2 pieces toast
1 teaspoon butter or margarine
1 orange
1 cup (8 ounces) milk

Snack
1 cup (8 ounces) low fat, fruit-flavored yogurt

Lunch
Healthy hummus pita:
  1/4 cup Healthy Hummus
    (see Recipes)
  1/2 cup salad greens
  1/2 tomato
  1/2 medium pita bread
    (2 ounces)
  1 1/2 ounces feta cheese
  2 tablespoons salad dressing
1 medium apple
1 ounce pretzels
1 cup (8 ounces) milk

Snack
4 graham cracker squares
1/2 cup (4 ounces) juice

Dinner
Pasta Salad, 1 serving (see
  Recipes)
1 cup cooked broccoli or carrots
2 teaspoons butter or margarine
1 cup (8 ounces) milk
Fresh fruit, your choice

Snack
Bread Pudding, 1 serving (see
  Recipes)

Day Two

Breakfast
1 cup high-fiber cereal
1 cup (8 ounces) milk
1 medium banana
1 slice whole grain toast with
  1 tablespoon peanut butter

Snack
1 piece fresh fruit or
1/4 cup dried fruit

Lunch
Chef's salad:
  2 cups salad greens
  1 cup raw sliced vegetables
  1 egg, cooked
  1 ounce Swiss cheese
  1–2 tablespoons salad dressing
1 large whole grain roll
  (2 ounces)
1 cup (8 ounces) milk
1 piece or 1/2 cup chopped fresh
  fruit

Snack
Bran and Molasses Muffin (see
  Recipes)

Dinner
Vegetarian Stew, 1 serving (see
  Recipes)
1 1/2 cups cooked rice
1–2 teaspoons butter or margarine
1 cup (8 ounces) milk

Snack
1 cup (8 ounces) plain, low-fat
  yogurt mixed with 1 teaspoon
  sugar, over 1 cup cubed fruit,
  topped with 1 ounce crunchy
  cereal

Day Three

Breakfast
Frozen Fruit Smoothie (see
  Recipes)

Snack
Bran and Molasses Muffin (see
  Recipes)
1–2 teaspoons butter or margarine

Lunch
Vegetarian Stew topped with 1
  ounce sharp cheddar cheese
  (see Recipes)
1 cup cooked rice
1 teaspoon butter or margarine
1 cup (8 ounces) milk
1 piece fresh fruit

Snack
Healthy Hummus, 1/4 cup (see
  Recipes)
1/2 cup raw vegetables

Dinner
Zucchini Frittata, 1 serving (see
  Recipes)
2 ounces French bread
1 cup cooked vegetables
1 teaspoon butter or margarine
1 piece fresh fruit

Snack
2 small oatmeal raisin cookies
1/2 cup (4 ounces) milk

Appendix 3

Delicious and Nutritious Recipes

WHEN YOU'RE EXPECTING a baby, it pays to have healthy recipes for easy-to-make fare on hand. Use the following 10 recipes to get started with healthy ways to prepare meals and snacks that are good sources of important nutrients during pregnancy. For example, Angel Hair with Clam Sauce is packed with iron; Frozen Fruit Smoothie provides a healthy dose of calcium; and Vegetarian Stew is a winner for folate.

Angel Hair with Clam Sauce
Serves 2

> 6 ounces angel hair pasta
> 3 tablespoons olive oil
> 4 cloves garlic, minced
> 2 6 1/2-ounce cans minced clams, undrained
> Salt and freshly ground black pepper to taste
> 2 rounded tablespoons flavored dry breadcrumbs
> 2 tablespoons chopped fresh parsley

1. Cook pasta according to package directions.

2. While pasta is cooking, heat 2 tablespoons olive oil over medium heat in a large skillet. Add garlic and cook for about one minute (do not let garlic become browned).

3. Stir in clams and liquid from can. Simmer for about 2 minutes. Season with pepper and salt if desired.

4. In a small saucepan, heat 1 tablespoon olive oil over medium heat. Add breadcrumbs and stir until golden, about 2 to 3 minutes.

5. Drain pasta and add to skillet with clam sauce, mixing until pasta is coated. Serve sprinkled with breadcrumbs and parsley.

Per serving: 598 calories; 34 grams protein; 17 grams fat; 2 grams fiber; 110 milligrams calcium; 25 milligrams iron; 480 milligrams sodium; 15 micrograms folate.

Frozen Fruit Smoothie

Serves 1

> 1/2 cup frozen fruit, such as berries or banana chunks
>
> 1 cup low-fat lemon yogurt
>
> 1/2 cup calcium-fortified orange juice

Mix all ingredients in a blender or food processor until smooth.

Per serving: 387 calories; 14 grams protein; 3 grams fat; 2 grams fiber; 708 milligrams calcium; 0 iron; 163 milligrams sodium; 110 micrograms folate.

Vegetarian Stew

Serves 6

> 2 tablespoons vegetable oil
>
> 3 carrots, diced
>
> 3 celery stalks, diced
>
> 2 medium onions, diced
>
> 10 cloves garlic, minced
>
> 4 cups chopped zucchini
>
> 1 cup peeled and chopped eggplant
>
> 1 cup water
>
> 1 28-ounce can whole tomatoes
>
> 1 10-ounce package fresh spinach, washed and cleaned
>
> 2 19-ounce cans garbanzo beans, drained
>
> 2 teaspoons dried parsley
>
> 1 teaspoon dried thyme
>
> 1 teaspoon dried rosemary
>
> Salt and pepper to taste

1. Heat oil in a large soup pot over medium high heat.

2. Add the carrots, celery, onions, and garlic. Cook until the onions are translucent.

3. Add the zucchini and eggplant. Cook for 5 to 7 minutes.

4. Add water and continue to cook for about 5 minutes. Add tomatoes and their juice, spinach, and garbanzo beans. Bring the mixture to a boil. Season with herbs; add salt and pepper to taste. Serve over rice or pasta.

Per serving: 298 calories; 14 grams protein; 8 grams fat; 14 grams fiber; 169 milligrams calcium; 5 milligrams iron; 515 milligrams sodium; 245 micrograms folate.

Chicken and Apples
Serves 4

> 3 tablespoons vegetable oil, divided
> 1 pound skinless, boneless chicken breast, cut into 1-inch cubes
> 2 medium red bell peppers, chopped
> 2 medium onions, chopped
> 1 cup chopped celery (about 3 stalks)
> 2 Golden Delicious apples, cored and sliced
> 2 tablespoons cornstarch
> 1/2 cup apple juice
> 3 tablespoons cider vinegar
> 3 tablespoons soy sauce

1. Stir-fry chicken in large nonstick skillet with 1 tablespoon oil until cooked through (no longer pink). Remove from pan and cover to keep warm.

2. Add vegetables to skillet along with 2 tablespoons oil. Cook until tender, about 3–5 minutes.

3. Return chicken to pan. Add apples and stir until heated through.

4. Combine the remaining ingredients in a small bowl. Add to chicken, vegetable, and apple mixture. Cook until sauce thickens, about 5 minutes.

Per serving: 345 calories; 33 grams protein; 12 grams fat; 5 grams fiber; 44 milligrams calcium; 2 milligrams iron; 872 milligrams sodium; 42 micrograms folate.

Beef Wraps

Serves 4

> 1 pound extra lean ground beef
>
> 1 tablespoon chili powder (if desired)
>
> Salt and pepper to taste
>
> 1 10-ounce package frozen chopped spinach, thawed and well drained
>
> 1 1/4 cups salsa
>
> 3/4 cup shredded cheddar cheese
>
> 8 6-inch corn tortillas

1. Brown ground beef over medium heat until no longer pink. Pour off drippings.

2. Season beef with chili powder, and salt and pepper to taste.

3. Stir in spinach and salsa. Cook over medium heat until heated through.

4. Remove from heat and stir in the cheese. To serve, place 1/2 cup beef in the center of each tortilla and roll up.

Per serving: 500 calories; 32 grams protein; 28 grams fat; 6 grams fiber; 368 milligrams calcium; 5 milligrams iron; 552 milligrams sodium; 115 micrograms folate.

Pasta Salad

Serves 6

> 1 cup orzo, or other small pasta
>
> 2 tablespoons olive oil
>
> 3 tablespoons lemon juice
>
> 1/4 teaspoon black pepper
>
> 12 ounces artichoke hearts, drained
>
> 1 19-ounce can chickpeas, rinsed and drained
>
> 4 ounces feta cheese, crumbled
>
> 1 1/2 cups 1% low-fat cottage cheese
>
> 1 teaspoon dried dill
>
> 2 large tomatoes, chopped

1. Cook orzo according to package directions. Transfer to colander and drain thoroughly.

2. In a large bowl, combine orzo with remaining ingredients. Toss gently.

3. Serve immediately or chill for later use.

Per serving: 307 calories; 18 grams protein; 11 grams fat; 6 grams fiber; 167 milligrams calcium; 3 milligrams iron; 626 milligrams sodium; 83 micrograms folate.

Zucchini Frittata
Serves 4

5 eggs

Salt and pepper to taste

1 teaspoon dried basil

1 cup 1% low-fat cottage cheese

5 tablespoons grated Parmesan cheese

2 tablespoons olive oil

1 large tomato, chopped

1 medium zucchini, washed, halved lengthwise, and thinly sliced

1. In a medium bowl, beat eggs lightly with salt, pepper, and basil. Stir in cottage cheese and half the Parmesan cheese. Set aside.

2. In a 12-inch nonstick skillet, lightly saute tomatoes and zucchini in the olive oil until zucchini is lightly browned.

3. Pour in egg mixture, and sprinkle with remaining Parmesan cheese. Cook over medium-low heat until eggs are well set, about 20 minutes.

4. Cut into 4 wedges, and serve immediately.

Per serving: 249 calories; 18 grams protein; 15 grams fat; 1 gram fiber; 155 milligrams calcium; 1 milligram iron; 351 milligrams sodium; 23 micrograms folate.

Healthy Hummus
Makes 2 cups

4 cloves garlic, peeled and minced

1 medium onion, peeled and chopped

1 teaspoon sesame oil plus 2 tablespoons

1 19-ounce can garbanzo beans, drained (about 2 cups)

1/4 cup minced fresh parsley or 1 tablespoon dried parsley

2 tablespoons lemon juice

1/4 teaspoon salt

1/4 teaspoon ground cumin

1/4 teaspoon hot sauce (optional)

1. Saute garlic and onion in 1 teaspoon sesame oil over low to medium heat in a nonstick skillet.

2. Transfer garlic and onion mixture to food processor. Add remaining ingredients and process until smooth.

3. Transfer to a small bowl, cover, and chill 1 hour.

4. Serve as a dip with raw vegetables or use as sandwich or cracker spread.

Per 2 tablespoon serving: 108 calories; 4 grams protein; 5 grams fat; 3 grams fiber; 23 milligrams calcium; 1 milligram iron; 244 milligrams sodium; 23 micrograms folate.

Per 1/4 cup serving: 216 calories; 8 grams protein; 10 grams fat; 6 grams fiber; 46 milligrams calcium; 2 milligrams iron; 488 milligrams sodium; 46 micrograms folate.

Bread Pudding

Serves 8

> 1 cup sugar
>
> 1 teaspoon nutmeg
>
> 2 cups 2% reduced-fat milk
>
> 1 teaspoon vanilla
>
> 2 eggs
>
> 2 1/2 cups stale, or toasted, French bread cubes
>
> 1 cup raisins

1. Heat oven to 350 degrees F. Grease a 2-quart baking dish.

2. In large bowl, combine first five ingredients; mix until smooth.

3. Fold in bread cubes and raisins. Pour mixture into prepared baking dish.

4. Bake for 45 minutes to 1 hour, or until knife inserted in center comes out clean. Cool slightly and serve. Or refrigerate for later use.

Per serving: 247 calories; 5 grams protein; 3 grams fat; 2 grams fiber; 97 milligrams calcium; 1 milligram iron; 134 milligrams sodium; 78 micrograms folate.

Bran and Molasses Muffins

Makes 12 muffins

2 cups shreds of whole bran cereal with extra fiber

1 1/2 cups skim milk

1/4 cup molasses

1/2 cup oil

1 egg

1 1/2 cups all-purpose flour

1/2 cup sugar

1 1/2 teaspoons baking soda

1/4 teaspoon salt

1/2 teaspoon cinnamon

1/2 cup raisins or other dried fruit, chopped

1. Heat oven to 400 degrees F. Grease 12 muffin cups or line with paper baking cups.

2. Combine cereal, milk, and molasses in a medium bowl. Let stand 2 minutes or until cereal is soft.

3. Add oil and egg to the cereal mixture and beat well. Set aside.

4. In a large bowl, combine flour, sugar, baking soda, salt, and cinnamon and mix well. Stir in the dried fruit.

5. Add softened cereal mixture and stir just until dry ingredients are moistened. Do not overmix.

6. Divide batter among the muffin cups. Bake for 15 to 17 minutes or until toothpick inserted in center comes out clean. Remove from pan, and cool slightly.

Per muffin: 201 calories; 5 grams protein; 6 grams fat; 6 grams fiber; 97 milligrams calcium; 3 milligrams iron; 381 milligrams sodium; 38 micrograms folate.

Index

acesulfame-K, 8
adolescents
  caloric recommenda-
    tions for, 3
  recommended servings,
    36
  weight gain recom-
    mendations, 2
alcohol consumption, viii,
  ix, x, 32
allergies, milk, 23
American College of
  Obstetricians and
  Gynecologists
  (ACOG), 2, 45, 65
anemia
  iron-deficiency, 24–25,
    59
  and vegetarianism,
    59
  megaloblastic, 17
Angel Hair with Clam
  Sauce, 75–76
appointments, prenatal,
  scheduling of, viii
artificial sweeteners,
  safety of, 8
aspartame, safety of, 8
aversions, food, 52

B vitamins, 17–18
  folate, viii, 17–18
  thiamin, 17
Beef Wraps, 78
beverages, viii, 6, 29–33
  alcohol, 30
  caffeinated, 30–31
  decaffeinated, 32
  and exercise, 46–47
  herbal tea, 32
  recommended intake,
    29
birth defects
  and caffeine, 30
  fetal alcohol syndrome,
    32
  spina bifida, viii

and high vitamin A
  intakes, 16
birthweight, 1
blood cholesterol, 11
blood disorders
  iron-deficiency anemia,
    24–25, 59
  megaloblastic anemia,
    17
blood pressure, role of
  sodium, 25
body temperature, regu-
  lating during exercise,
    46–47
Bran and Molasses
  Muffins, 81
Bread Pudding, 80
bread, cereal, rice, and
  pasta group, 5, 36, 37,
    67
breakfast ideas, 40–41
breast-feeding
  caloric needs for, ix,
    36, 61–62
  recommended caffeine
    intake, 30–31
  recommended sodium
    intake, 26
  and weight loss, 61–62

caffeine, viii, 30–31
  reducing intake, 31
  sources of, 31
calcium, ix, x, 20–24
  recommended intake,
    20
  role of, 20
  effects of sodium, 26
  sources, 21
  supplements, 22
  and vegetarianism, 58
calories
  budgeting of, 3–4, 5
  recommended intakes,
    ix, 3, 36
  for breast-feeding,
    61–62

for non-breast-feed-
  ing women,
    62–63
carbohydrate-rich foods, 6
carbohydrates, 5–8
  caloric contents of, 6
  categories of, 6
  as energy source, 5, 6
  cereals, fortified breakfast,
    6
cheeses, soft, safety concerns for, 56
Chicken and Apples, 77
cholesterol, blood, 11
coffee consumption, viii,
  30–31
  effects on iron intake,
    24
comfrey, 28
constipation, x, 51, 53
  and iron supplements,
    24
cravings, food, 3

dairy products, 20–24, 36,
  38–39, 68–79
  allergies, 23
  and lactose intolerance,
    22–23
  increasing intakes of,
    23–24
  recommended intakes,
    x, 38–39, 68–79
decaffeinated beverages,
  32
dehydration, and caffeine,
  30
development, fetus, 1–4
  and alcohol consump-
    tion, 32
  and dietary supple-
    ments, 27
diabetes, gestational, 60
dietitian, registered, ix, 22
drug use, illicit, viii

echinacia, 28